D1435568

BRAIN
BOOSTING
FOODS

JANET
MACCARO, PhD, CNC

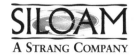

A STRANG COMPANY

Most Strang Communications/Charisma House/Siloam/FrontLine/Excel Books/Realms products are available at special quantity discounts for bulk purchase for sales promotions, premiums, fund-raising, and educational needs. For details, write Strang Communications/Charisma House/Siloam/FrontLine/ Excel Books/Realms, 600 Rinehart Road, Lake Mary, Florida 32746, or telephone (407) 333-0600.

Brain-Boosting Foods by Janet Maccaro
Published by Siloam
A Strang Company
600 Rinehart Road
Lake Mary, Florida 32746
www.siloam.com

Cover Designer: Judith McKittrick
Design Director: Bill Johnson
Author Photograph © Markow Southwest, www.paulmarkow.com

Library of Congress Cataloging-in-Publication Data:

Maccaro, Janet C.
  Brain-boosting foods / Janet Maccaro.
    p. cm.
  Includes bibliographical references (p.   ).
  ISBN 978-1-59979-225-5
  1. Brain. 2. Nutrition. 3. Human behavior--Nutritional aspects. 4. Brain chemistry. I. Title.
  QP376.M115 2008
  612.8--dc22
                              2008003297

Neither the publisher nor the author is engaged in rendering professional advice or services to the individual reader. The ideas, procedures, and suggestions in this book are not intended as a substitute for consulting with your physician. All matters regarding your health require medical supervision. Neither the author nor the publisher shall be liable or responsible for any loss or damage allegedly arising from any information or suggestion in this book.

While the author has made every effort to provide accurate telephone numbers and Internet addresses at the time of publication, neither the publisher nor the author assumes any responsibility for errors or for changes that occur after publication

08 09 10 11 12 — 987654321
Printed in the United States of America

CONTENTS

SECTION 4: REBUILDING YOUR BRAIN

SECTION 5: YOUR HEALTHY BRAIN

INTRODUCTION

Your brain weighs only about 3 pounds, and yet it is the control center of your body. It is the most amazingly complex organ that you possess. It controls not only the functions of each part of your body, but also your movements (both voluntary and involuntary) and your physical sensations. Your brain is also in charge of your emotions, both pleasurable and painful, and it governs your behaviors. By using your brain, you make all of your decisions, both large and small. It is responsible for all of your thought patterns.

Like your other organs, your brain is permeated with circulating blood and bathed in chemicals. It uses energy—lots of it. It can get sick. The smooth functioning of your brain depends on what happens to you and what you eat in the course of your daily life, and we're learning more about this all the time.

The big question I want to answer in this book is, are you feeding your brain the right foods? This is something over which most of us in the United States of America have some control. We are blessed with abundant resources. As we learn more about how to maintain healthy bodies—which includes having healthy brains—we can alter our nutritional habits and make changes in what kinds of foods we are eating and drinking. Aside from *not* taking mood-altering drugs, the most important determinant of your brain health is your nutrition and your accompanying activity level.

You can find out firsthand that certain foods make a *big* difference in how you feel and how well you can function.

It's good to become acquainted with as much information as possible about good nutrition. You decide what you want to try. See what works and what doesn't. Work toward that excellent balance of quality and quantity of foods, beverages, and supplements, along with balanced attention to other facets such as sleep and exercise.

You cannot expect your body to function optimally if you have not provided it with the right fuel. And if you have "let yourself go" to any degree through neglect, bad habits, or circumstances beyond your control such as illnesses or injuries, you may need to apply some extra effort to recovering the health you once had.

I have organized this book into five sections, each containing several short chapters. The sections cover these topics: "Nutrition and Brain Function," "Your Brain and Your Mental Health," "Your Brain and Your Physical Health," "Rebuilding Your Brain," and "Your Healthy Brain." Each of the fifty brief chapters includes several callouts that capture for you the key information from that chapter: "Basic Brain Food," "Supplemental Brain Food," and "Food for Thought." The last callout captures the best pieces of nutritional information from each chapter: one caution called "Brain-Busting Tip-Off" and one final "Brain-Boosting Tip."

It is my hope that this book can provide you with much help. I want you to combine what you learn about your physical, mental, and emotional health, and I want you to better understand how you can take care of the nutritional needs of your brain. Here's to your present and future brainpower and to all the great brain-boosting endeavors you will undertake!

SECTION 1

NUTRITION AND BRAIN FUNCTION

chapter 1

HOW WE'RE MADE 101

YOUR BRAIN IS especially sensitive to your diet, and the way it works reflects changes in what you consume.

[The brain] depends on a continuous supply of nutrients from the blood, some of which are synthesized in other organs of the body, such as choline [found in eggs]. Others, which cannot be synthesized in mammalian systems at all, are "essential" components that must be furnished by the diet. These essential nutrients include vitamins, amino acids and fatty acids....

Nutrition can alter brain function in short time frames, for example, by altering neurotransmitters and neuronal firing, and in the long-term, such as by altering membrane structure. The importance of proper nutrition during brain development has been appreciated for several decades. That the nutritional requirements of the brain of mature and aged individuals may differ from those of the young was established more recently. Genetics also affects dietary needs. Although classic vitamin and other nutritional "deficiencies" are major public health concerns in underdeveloped countries, they also occur in industrialized societies. Vitamin insufficiencies can occur secondary to alcohol or drug abuse or other psychiatric disorders, as a result of genetic variation or because particular age groups have special requirements. Nutritional therapy...may eventually provide a productive approach to the treatment of common adult neurodegenerative disorders, such as Alzheimer's and Parkinson's diseases, that encompass complex interactions of genetics and the environment.[1]

Your brain is amazing! It communicates with the rest of your body through your nervous system. Nerves send messages up and down your spinal cord and out to the ends of your fingertips and toes. Neurons are the cells of your nervous system, and each one looks like an octopus. These branching neurons send the signals from one to another almost instantaneously, and they can "learn" specific patterns and pathways to follow.

Let's begin by discussing the four main building blocks of good brain health. They are:

- Fatty acids (such as omega-3 fats from fish and nuts)
- Amino acids (from proteins)
- Glucose (from carbohydrates)
- Micronutrients (such as antioxidants, vitamins, and minerals from fresh fruit and vegetables)

Put simply, fatty acids help form your brain, amino acids keep neurotransmitters running smoothly, a steady supply of glucose gives it fuel, and micronutrients protect it.

To break it down even further, researchers have learned which micronutrients and chemical compounds are the most important for the healthy growth and functioning of the brain and nervous system. Some of them can be manufactured in our bodies, such as vitamin D (which only requires a little sunshine, although some of our foods also supply it). Our bodies can't manufacture most of them—we need to open our mouths and chew and swallow or drink the nutrients that we need. That is the reason for the recommended daily allowance of some vitamins and minerals. For instance, a major deficiency in vitamin B_{12} or iron can inhibit our brain functions by impairing the connections between the nerve fibers. Without peak brain function, we cannot adequately process the information that comes to us through our senses.

Here's the simple fact about your incredibly complex body and brain: what you eat—or don't eat—makes a significant impact on your quality of life.

BASIC BRAIN FOOD

To function well, your brain needs good food.

SUPPLEMENTAL BRAIN FOOD

Take your daily multivitamin.

FOOD FOR THOUGHT

BRAIN-BUSTING TIP-OFF # 1: Just a little nutritional information is not enough.

BRAIN-BOOSTING TIP # 1: A smart start to a better brain is eating choline-rich eggs.

chapter 2

FROM THE WOMB...

WHEN A WOMAN is pregnant, what she eats is one of the most important influences on the health of her developing baby. Nutritional deficiencies do not have a mere temporary effect on the mother's own health; they can have a permanent effect on the baby's health, even causing life-shortening disabilities such as developmental delay and cerebral palsy. Less serious disabilities are also permanent: learning disabilities, sight and hearing difficulties, and more.

Even before a woman becomes pregnant, she should prepare herself nutritionally. One of the most important vitamins to take is folic acid, which is one of the B vitamins. Having enough folic acid daily can help to prevent serious birth defects of a baby's brain and spine. Such birth defects develop so early in a pregnancy that most women do not even realize they are pregnant yet.

Does this mean pregnant women should take vitamin supplements? Yes, but they shouldn't overdo it. A good prenatal multivitamin supplement is needed every day, but eating a balanced, healthy diet is equally important.

What should be included in a pregnant woman's daily diet? For starters, at least seven servings of fruits and vegetables, along with six to nine modest servings of whole-grain breads and cereals.[1] Beyond that, every pregnant woman should consume at least four servings of dairy products every day in order to obtain the calcium she and her growing baby require for strong bones and teeth. (Pregnant women should have at least 1,000 mg of calcium daily, which often involves taking a calcium supplement.) If a woman is lactose-intolerant, other calcium-containing nondairy foods should be established as part of her daily menu.[2]

A pregnant woman's protein needs are about 10 grams per day higher than the protein needs of other people, or about 60 grams of protein per day. However, most American diets are fairly high in protein, so the only adjustments needed may involve the choices of protein sources. Fish, while providing a natural source of omega-3 fatty acids, have been implicated in mercury-related problems. Sixty grams of protein can come from as little as two (well-cooked) servings of lean meat, fish, or poultry, plus nuts, dried beans, and eggs. Protein builds muscle, tissue, enzymes, hormones, and antibodies for both the mother and her baby. Protein-rich foods also contain B vitamins and iron, which are very important for the mother's blood.[3] In addition, expectant mothers should not forget to drink plenty of clean water, which is always important to overall health.

The old saying says that a pregnant woman should "eat for two." This isn't strictly true. In fact, if she eats twice as much food, she will gain too much weight. A pregnant woman's body only requires about 300 extra calories a day. But it is certainly true from the point of view of nutritional quality. Every pregnant woman should know—and follow—established guidelines for her daily diet. This is not a time for her to indulge her sweet tooth or fill up on her favorite foods. The all-important physical and mental development and health of her baby is at stake.

BASIC BRAIN FOOD

Pregnant women: your baby's healthy development depends on your diet.

SUPPLEMENTAL BRAIN FOOD

Pregnant women should take a prenatal vitamin that contains folic acid.

FOOD FOR THOUGHT

BRAIN-BUSTING TIP-OFF #2: Pregnant women should not eat undercooked meats!

BRAIN-BOOSTING TIP #2: Pregnant women are nourishing two brains and should eat 60 grams of protein daily.

chapter 3

CHILD'S PLAY

FROM BIRTH, THE growth and health of your child's brain and body depend upon a combination of factors, and your child's diet is one of the most important ones.

A research report sums it up: human development hinges on the interactions between nature and nurture.

- How humans develop and learn depends critically and continually on the interactions between nature (an individual's genetic endowment) and nurture (the nutrition, surroundings, care, stimulation, and teaching that are provided or withheld).
- The impact of environmental factors on the young child's brain development is dramatic and specific, not merely influencing the general direction of development, but actually affecting how the intricate circuitry of the human brain is "wired."[1]

Again, we see that without good nutrition, the healthy development of your child's "control central"—his or her brain—is compromised. The first three years of your child's life are vital. Poor nutrition during those critical years can permanently cripple not only physical growth but also brain structure and function. In other words, even if caloric intake is adequate, less-than-adequate *nutritional* intake can hamper your child's mental development in ways that cannot be overcome later in life.

One logical and natural solution to the nutritional challenge is for mothers to breast-feed their infants for at least the first six months of their lives if at all possible. Breast milk is the perfect food for fast-growing little bodies and minds. It contains the right balance of nutrients in the most digestible form to help an infant become a strong toddler. The proteins, calcium, and iron in breast milk are more easily absorbed than those in formula or cow's milk. The fats, vitamins, and carbohydrates in breast milk are exactly what a newborn needs. Many components of breast milk can help protect a child from diseases and infections, including E coli and salmonella. Along with the antibodies, enzymes, and hormones, none of which can be added to even the best infant formula, they help make breast milk the ideal "brain food" for infancy.[2]

As solid foods are introduced (between four and six months, depending on your child's ability to sit up and hold up his or her head, and the ability to reject or accept food from a small spoon), you should start by introducing rice cereal, which provides the fewest allergic responses. One serving of a new food should be very small—only a couple of teaspoons. One food should be introduced at a time, allowing a week between new types of food. The foods should be as smooth and easy to swallow as possible.[3] To minimize allergies, wait until after your child's first birthday to introduce eggs, citrus fruits and juices, cow's milk, or honey. Avoid seafood, peanuts, and tree nuts altogether before your child reaches the age of two or three.[4]

Soon your infant is well on the way to becoming a lively, healthy toddler who can enjoy all kinds of healthy foods for the rest of his or her life.

BASIC BRAIN FOOD

Breast-feeding provides the best start for your baby.

SUPPLEMENTAL BRAIN FOOD

Provide your baby with infant cereals that are fortified with iron and B vitamins.

FOOD FOR THOUGHT

BRAIN-BUSTING TIP-OFF #3: Do not let your baby drink sugary juices.

BRAIN-BOOSTING TIP #3: The nutrients, antibodies, enzymes, and hormones in breast milk make it the best "brain food" for your baby.

chapter 4

NUTRITIONAL BALANCE = BRAIN BALANCE

MOVING FROM CHILDHOOD back to adulthood, I want to lay some more groundwork for talking about the importance of brain foods. It would be impossible to minimize the importance of the role good nutrition plays in your overall health and body balance. Nutritional balance equals body balance, which equals brain balance.

Your body uses the nutrition with which you supply it to build, maintain, and repair your tissues. Nutrients empower your cells to relay messages back and forth to conduct essential chemical reactions that enable you to think, see, hear, smell, taste, move, breathe, and eliminate waste.

Human beings share the same basic physical makeup, but each of us is as individual as our thumbprint when it comes to our specific nutritional needs. Many factors combine to determine your individual nutritional needs, including the amount of stress you experience and how you manage it, how your hectic lifestyle depletes your nutritional storehouse, what your dietary habits are, and whether you are overly acidic or overly alkaline.

What do I mean by "acidic" and "alkaline"? In childhood, most of us are naturally alkaline, and this is true into our teens and early adulthood. But by the fourth decade of life, most of us become overly acidic because of our exposure to stress, poor food selections, and environmental toxins. Being overly acidic makes you susceptible to many ailments, including headaches, chronic illnesses, colds and flu, digestive problems, urinary tract infections, and chronic fatigue. Having a healthy acid/alkaline balance means you enjoy mental clarity, fast recovery from illness and injury, vitality, and energy. The good news is that you can bring your system into a more balanced state by eating foods that will turn acidic conditions around.

The following foods should become the centerpiece of your daily regimen:

- *Legumes*: baked beans, kidney beans, lima beans, soybeans, tofu, chickpeas, black beans
- *Grains*: brown rice, barley, oats, rye, millet, quinoa, hominy grits, buckwheat
- *Poultry/eggs*: free-range chicken, duck, turkey, egg yolk, whole eggs
- *Meat*: fish, shellfish, tofu (preferred over red meat and pork)
- *Condiments*: hot peppers, garlic, canned olives, flax meal, kelp
- *Sweeteners*: blackstrap molasses, honey, brown rice syrup or maple syrup
- *Vegetables*: pumpkin, sweet peppers, spinach, carrots, squash, asparagus, turnips, cabbage, broccoli, sweet potatoes, onions, peas, celery, corn, lettuce, mushrooms, brussels sprouts
- *Unsweetened fruits*: figs, papayas, persimmons, dates, cantaloupes, melons
- *Nuts and seeds*: walnuts, almonds, flaxseeds, hazelnuts, pecans, poppy seeds, pumpkin seeds, sesame seeds, sunflower seeds
- *Beverages*: mineral water, distilled water, herbal or green tea, soy or rice milk

If you are overly acidic, you will feel better if you consume more complex carbohydrates in your daily diet. If you are a high alkaline producer, you will feel better if your diet contains more proteins. By complex carbohydrates, I mean a combination of whole grains and legumes. I recommend fish and poultry over red meats for both metabolic types because they are lower in unhealthy saturated fat, and they contain a full spectrum of essential amino acids as well as being great sources for vitamins E, D, and A. Fish provide omega-3 fatty acids that fight inflammation and reduce your chances of suffering a stroke.

Fresh fruit has an alkalizing effect on the body and is extremely high in vitamins and nutrients. Natural fruit sugar (from fresh fruit only) is easily transformed into quick, nonfattening energy, which speeds up your metabolism. Fresh fruits also have the benefit of adding fiber and fluid to your system. For the best energy conversion and cleansing benefits, fruits should be eaten before noon. To help all your body processes, be sure to drink plenty of water.

Pay attention to your own personal body chemistry and you will not regret it.

BASIC BRAIN FOOD

Are you acidic or alkaline? Learn more about your own personal body chemistry, and adjust your nutritional intake accordingly.

SUPPLEMENTAL BRAIN FOOD

Consider taking supplemental digestive enzymes if you don't seem to be able to derive enough benefit from the food you eat.

FOOD FOR THOUGHT

BRAIN-BUSTING TIP-OFF #4: Coffee and black tea are acidic even if decaffeinated.

BRAIN-BOOSTING TIP #4: For simple brain nutrition, think "complex"— complex carbohydrates such as whole grains and legumes.

chapter 5

NOURISH YOUR BRAIN:
GABA AND MAGNESIUM

Y OUR BRAIN IS one of God's most extraordinary creations. It houses and expresses your personality, the information you have learned, your past memories, and your future desires. It coordinates your consciousness with your unconsciousness, and it gives your life impetus and purpose. Using your brain, you can read this book and then go to the kitchen to prepare your next meal. You can get to know what foods your *brain* desires and requires, and what kinds of special treatment it requires for top functioning.

GABA (gamma-aminobutyric acid) is a naturally occurring amino acid. It is the main inhibitory neurotransmitter that restores your brain, regulating anxiety, moods, muscle spasms, depression, and chronic stress. For its proper metabolism, other nutrients work along with GABA, in particular, magnesium. Since GABA actually fills the GABA receptor sites in the brain, while mood-altering drugs merely attach to the receptors, proponents believe that by restoring the brain chemistry with GABA and other amino acids, the brain becomes balanced so that sensory reception is sharp, clear, and intact.

Trauma and stress deplete your GABA. Emotions such as grief, anger, fear, and anxiety, as well as physical pain, all play a big part in this depletion. When your GABA supply has been depleted, your entire body will tell you about it. Your eyes will dilate and your vision will blur; your mouth will be dry; your heart will race; the bronchioles of your lungs will constrict; your stomach will contract and make digestion difficult and you will need to make frequent trips to the bathroom; and your adrenal glands will pump out adrenaline, leaving you weak. If left unresolved, you may develop chronic pains, insomnia, panic attacks, headaches, and emotional discomfort.

Magnesium is a vital mineral, enhancing the action and effect of amino acids. Therefore, you need to find out if you need more of it. The symptoms of magnesium deficiency are the same as those that occur with anxiety, stress, and emotional depletion. They include depression, fatigue, irregular heartbeat, irritable bowel syndrome and spastic symptoms, headaches, noise sensitivity, fibromyalgia, low blood sugar, dizziness, constipation, asthma, and chronic pain.

To turn around a depletion of magnesium, add the following foods to your daily diet: almonds, blackberries, broccoli, green beans, kidney beans, navy beans, soybeans, watermelon, bananas, black-eyed peas, dates, kasha (buckwheat), millet, shrimp, and tuna. Even if you eat foods that are rich in magnesium, you may require magnesium supplementation because chronic stress makes your blood pressure increase, which causes magnesium to be released from your blood cells into your blood plasma, after which it is excreted in your urine.

In your body, GABA is manufactured in conjunction with B-vitamin compounds, especially vitamin B_6. Therefore, it is a good idea to nourish your body and brain with foods that are high in both protein and vitamin B_6, such as fish (particularly mackerel) and wheat bran. (Research is conflicting regarding good food sources of GABA.[1])

The best idea is to take a good GABA supplement.

BASIC BRAIN FOOD

Stress and emotions such as grief, anger, fear, and anxiety play a big part in depleting your body of GABA.

SUPPLEMENTAL BRAIN FOOD

If you suffer from the symptoms above, supplement your diet with GABA and magnesium.

FOOD FOR THOUGHT

Brain-Busting Tip-Off #5: Don't let stress drive you to junk foods. Now is when you need the best nutrition you can get.

Brain-Boosting Tip #5: To help diffuse stress and its effects on your brain, go for fish, beans, kasha, millet, blackberries, broccoli, bananas, dates, watermelon, and almonds.

chapter 6

FISH = BRAIN FOOD

A s I MENTIONED in chapter 1, amino acids from proteins are one of the main building blocks for boosting your brain. Proteins are made from chains of amino acids, and proteins are found in every tissue of your body. Muscles, organs, glands, cell membranes, enzymes, and neurotransmitters are all proteins. If you were to take the water and fat out of your body, 75 percent of what would remain would be protein. Every living cell in your body contains and is maintained by protein, as well as all of your body fluids except bile and urine. Amino acids are responsible for the growth, repair, and maintenance of your body, and, most importantly, they are sources of energy that play a vital role in the way your brain functions.

Amino acids heal and restore brain function because they control the anxiety stop switch, they function as a muscle relaxant, and they act as pain relievers. More importantly, as I mentioned in the previous chapter, amino acids create new neurotransmitters for proper brain communication, helping you to think better, feel better, and stay healthy.

Your body depends on the twenty-plus different types of amino acids, and together they form over a thousand basic proteins. Your body can manufacture some of these amino acids, but nine essential amino acids must be obtained from food. Therefore, for optimal brain and body functioning, you need to be sure that your daily diet includes sources of protein, both incomplete sources (which supply some of the necessary amino acids) and sources of complete protein such as all types of meats and other animal products.

As an adult, you need to eat 7 to 9 grams of protein daily for every 20 pounds of body weight.[1] You can get this from complete sources or from incomplete sources that have been well combined. In most cases, a simple American diet furnishes more than enough protein. All you need is a bowl of breakfast cereal plus milk, a peanut butter and jelly sandwich for lunch, and a piece of fish with some beans for supper, and you have consumed about 70 grams of protein, which is more than enough for the average adult.[2] Six ounces of cooked fish provides 41.2 grams of high-quality protein. A half a cup of cooked kidney beans provides 7.6 grams of incomplete protein.[3] This is why your mother used to tell you that fish was a "brain food."

Choose a variety of low-fat sources of protein daily and eat modest servings. A normal serving of lean meat, poultry, or fish is 2 or 3 ounces in weight (about the size of a pack of playing cards). An average portion size for cooked dry legumes or beans is half a cup. One egg and 2 tablespoons of peanut butter count as 1 ounce of lean meat.

A healthy brain, well-supplied with amino acids, will stay conditioned and quick. Part of the health of your brain involves your mental and emotional health as well, and amino acids/proteins play a major role. Nutritional health practitioners can help you decide if you need to supplement the proteins you are able to obtain from food sources. Supplementation can be combined to match your personal needs. For instance, the following amino acid supplements may help to restore and replenish your brain:

- *Glutamine* helps to improve memory, recall, concentration, and alertness, and also helps to reduce sugar and alcohol cravings and control hypoglycemic reactions.
- *Lysine* is a natural treatment of hypothyroidism, Alzheimer's disease, and Parkinson's disease.
- *Tyrosine* converts in the body to the amino acid L-dopa. Helps to build the body's natural supply of adrenaline and thyroid hormones. It is also an antioxidant and a source of quick energy, especially for the brain. It is helpful for Parkinson's disease, depression, and hypertension. (Avoid tyrosine if you have cancerous melanoma or manic depression.)
- *Glycine* converts to creatine in the body to retard nerve and muscle degeneration. It helps to release growth hormones when taken in large doses, and it controls and regulates hypoglycemic symptoms, especially when taken in the morning upon rising.
- *Taurine* is a neurotransmitter that helps control the nervous system and hyperactivity. It helps to prevent

circulatory and heart disorders and helps to lower cholesterol. Natural sources are hard to find, so supplementation
is the best way to receive adequate amounts for therapeutic benefit.

In short, take advantage of amino acids. Amino acids are natural
tranquilizers!

BASIC BRAIN FOOD

Eat at least 7 to 9 grams of protein daily for each 20 pounds of your
body weight.

SUPPLEMENTAL BRAIN FOOD

Consider amino acid supplementation for optimal health.

FOOD FOR THOUGHT

BRAIN-BUSTING TIP-OFF #6: Don't skimp on protein in your diet, but
don't overdo it either.

BRAIN-BOOSTING TIP #6: To keep your brain's neurotransmitters
running at peak performance, eat a variety of fish often.

chapter 7

ANTIOXIDANTS AND YOUR BRAIN

THE CELLS OF your body are composed of molecules, and, as you may remember from high school, molecules consist of one or more atoms, with each proton nucleus being orbited by a number of electrons. Atoms are always seeking to achieve a state of maximum stability by gaining or losing electrons or by sharing electrons with other atoms. When weakened atoms split, they create odd, unpaired electrons, and free radicals are formed. Unstable free radicals try to capture their needed electrons from other compounds to gain stability. They usually attack the nearest stable molecule to "rob" it of an electron, which means that the second molecule now becomes a free radical. This process keeps happening until something stops it, and much damage can be done to cells in the process.

In your body, free radicals arise during normal body metabolic processes, but environmental factors such as tobacco smoke, herbicides, radiation, and pollution can hasten their formation. Naturally, free-radical damage becomes more noticeable as a person ages. The only way to retard free-radical damage is to provide the body with antioxidants, which are able to "donate" one of their own electrons without becoming unstable free radicals themselves. Vitamins E and C are especially effective in this regard. In essence, they help to prevent cell and therefore tissue damage that could otherwise lead to serious disease and functional difficulties.[1]

As your brain "fires" all day and all night, each of your billions of brain cells has more potential than other cells in your body for free-radical damage. You don't want the damage to occur at a faster rate than it can be repaired, or diminished brain function will be the result, somewhat like "rusting out."

In foods, antioxidants can often be identified by their bright colors, which is why you are often told to choose an array of colors of fresh produce. Those bright red cherries and tomatoes; orange carrots; yellow corn and mangos; and dark bluish purple blueberries, blackberries, and grapes abound with antioxidants.[2] The antioxidants that are found naturally in many foods, including fruits and vegetables, nuts, grains, and some meats, include:[3]

- Beta-carotene
- Lutein
- Lycopene
- Selenium
- Vitamin A
- Vitamin C
- Vitamin E

It's not a simple cause-and-effect equation. The more scientists research antioxidants, the more complex the story becomes. It isn't the case that massive doses of antioxidants will stave off all cancer, Alzheimer's disease, macular degeneration of the eye, or cardiovascular disease, but everyone can benefit from a healthy increase in his or her consumption of those bright-colored fresh fruits and vegetables.

What's the moral of the antioxidant story? The moral is: the older you are, the lower the level of antioxidants in your body and the more you need that fresh, unpeeled, organically grown apple instead of that piece of apple pie.

BASIC BRAIN FOOD

The more fruits and vegetables you eat, the healthier your cells will be.

SUPPLEMENTAL BRAIN FOOD

Take a good multivitamin supplement daily with additional vitamin C.

FOOD FOR THOUGHT

BRAIN-BUSTING TIP-OFF #7: There's no "magic antioxidant pill" that will eliminate all free-radical damage.

BRAIN-BOOSTING TIP #7: Brightly colored fruits and vegetables provide antioxidants that help protect your brain.

chapter 8

WATER: PURE AND ESSENTIAL

WATER MAKES UP more than 60 percent of your body and 75 percent of your brain. Your brain needs water to keep it functioning at high levels and to keep all of its circuits working. Dehydration depletes your brain of important fluids, and an article on the USDA Web site says:

> Research in young adults shows that mild dehydration corresponding to only 1–2 percent of body weight loss can lead to significant impairment in cognitive function. Dehydration in infants is associated with confusion, irritability, and lethargy. In children dehydration may produce decrements in cognitive performance.[1]

As an essential for your survival, water is second only to oxygen. Water helps to flush wastes and toxins, it regulates your body temperature, and it acts as a shock absorber for your joints, bones, and muscles. It cleanses your body inside and out. It transports nutrients, proteins, vitamins, minerals, and sugars for assimilation. When you drink enough water, you enable your brain and body to operate at peak performance.

The recommended amount of water consumption for the average person is eight to ten glasses per day. If this seems like a lot to you, just start slowly. Add a slice of fresh lemon, and you will get even more of a cleansing benefit.

Most of our municipal tap water is chlorinated, fluoridated, or treated to the point of becoming an irritant to the human system. Many toxic chemicals have found their way into the groundwater, adding more pollutants to our water supply. This growing concern about water purity has led to the huge bottled water industry. Stores today have whole aisles dedicated to bottled water.

Mineral water most often comes from natural springs with naturally occurring minerals and a taste that varies from one spring to the next. These naturally occurring minerals aid digestion and bowel function, and Europeans have long known its benefits. While distilled water is probably the purest water available, it has been demineralized, which is not ideal, especially in the long run. Sparkling water is naturally carbonated spring water that has usually had its carbonation boosted artificially as well. Many people maintain that a glass of sparkling water after dinner aids digestion. I advocate the use of a water filter on your kitchen sink faucet that will remove the impurities as the water flows out of the tap. Alternatively, use a water pitcher that contains a filter.

Whatever type of water you choose, the most important thing to remember is that you must pay conscious attention to getting your quota of water every day. Thirst is not a reliable signal that your body needs water. You can easily lose a quart or more of water during activity before you even feel thirsty. Do a simple test: if your urine color is dark yellow, start drinking more water. You will know that you are adequately hydrated when your urine becomes a pale straw color.

People in our society consume coffee by the gallon and soft drinks by the liter. Remember, caffeine and alcohol are diuretics; by making you lose water, they increase your need for water. Ideally, caffeine and alcohol do not belong in a health-building program.

BASIC BRAIN FOOD

Water is the most basic brain food of them all.

SUPPLEMENTAL BRAIN FOOD

Mineral water provides natural supplementation for you.

FOOD FOR THOUGHT

BRAIN-BUSTING TIP-OFF #8: Don't substitute caffeinated beverages for pure water.

BRAIN-BOOSTING TIP #8: Dehydration impairs cognitive function, so be sure to drink eight to ten glasses of water per day.

chapter 9

BUILDING LIFELONG
NUTRITIONAL HABITS

NUTRITION IS A vast and ever-expanding field. More research and discoveries are being made this minute, and it's impossible to keep up with everything. But we can agree on certain basics, and these will see us through. If we are already healthy and enjoy balanced brains and bodies, following the basics will keep us that way. If we are suffering from some depletion or debilitation, now's the time to learn about and establish good nutritional habits (along with good exercise and other good habits) in order to recover and then maintain the highest degree of health.

It's our brains that will help us know what to do. Our minds make us capable of both assimilating new information and using that information for decision making. What a sad thing it is when our overall health has declined to the degree that we can no longer make informed decisions about how to take care of ourselves. This can happen to anyone, and it may not be obvious. We live with so much advertising and societal pressure, and it gives us a false idea of nutritional health. We think we are doing great because we are enjoying our third latte of the day when really we're just wired from all that caffeine and so satiated we don't care to prepare ourselves a nutritionally balanced meal.

If you don't have a clue what to do, or if you experience compromised brain and body health but you don't know where to start, I want to offer you a leg up. Step up on the basics of brain-boosting health that you find in this book. Take my word for it—this works! If you don't know where to start, just take a chance and start *anywhere*, with something easy to do such as drinking more water, as was recommended in the previous chapter. Such a simple step as that may eliminate for you, as it has for many of my clients, all sorts of troubling physical and mental/emotional symptoms such as water retention and bloating, sluggish depression, and the inability to assimilate nutrients.

The nutritional basics always include *balance*. Your nutritional habits should enable you to eat, on a daily basis, from all of the six categories of nutrients that your body needs to acquire from food (you may remember that four of these are the main building blocks for your brain that we discussed in chapter 1):

- Protein
- Carbohydrates
- Fat
- Fiber
- Vitamins and minerals
- Water

The healthiest sources of these nutrients are low-fat animal products, whole grains, beans, nuts, and fresh fruits and vegetables. All of these brain-friendly foods will also help to prevent disease and promote health. Good nutrition supplies you with what your body and brain need to support healthy functioning. Good nutrition boosts all of the functions of your brain, which include governing your body functions and controlling your emotions.

It's never too late. Today, you can make good nutritional choices that will start to turn the health of your body and brain for the good.

BASIC BRAIN FOOD

Make intentional choices to establish lifelong nutritional habits.

SUPPLEMENTAL BRAIN FOOD

Every day, supplement your balanced diet with the extras that you cannot obtain from your "daily bread."

FOOD FOR THOUGHT

BRAIN-BUSTING TIP-OFF #9: Don't leave your nutritional choices to chance. Good nutritional habits do not happen automatically.

BRAIN-BOOSTING TIP #9: Brain-friendly foods include lean meat, whole grains, beans, nuts, fresh fruits, and veggies.

chapter 10

FILLING NUTRITIONAL GAPS: MAKING SUPPLEMENTS COUNT

FROM FOOD ALONE, no one can obtain all of the vitamins and minerals needed by his or her brain and body. Ideally, this would be possible, but our twenty-first-century methods of farming and marketing foods do not guarantee that you will get anywhere near the best nutritional value from the foods you buy at the supermarket.

That's why I wholeheartedly recommend dietary supplements to fill nutritional gaps in our daily diet. Even apart from modern farming and food-processing methods, illness, aging, and extreme diet practices may have put you in a spot where your body cannot absorb all of the nutrients you need from your food alone.

Understanding your daily supplemental needs will make for consistently vibrant brain health. Supplementing your diet with the correct amounts of the right nutrients will enhance the function of your immune system, your reproductive system, your digestive system, your circulatory system, and your nervous system (the home team working with those little gray cells). The right nutritional supplement protocol can help chase away fatigue, anxiety, headaches, depression, confusion, and memory loss, and can improve motor skills and concentration.

Maybe you have heard someone say, "Taking vitamins and supplements results only in expensive urine." The truth is, all substances are eventually excreted, but as your vitamins go on their way through your bloodstream, they build your health and enhance your life. Keeping your body blanketed with the full spectrum of vitamins and minerals is like having an insurance policy against decline in brain and body function.

Experts agree that one of the best ways to safeguard your health is to eat only the healthiest foods you can find. Plenty of fresh fruits, vegetables, and whole grains, along with low-fat dairy products, are the basic recommendations. This is because of all of the *phytochemicals*, or vitamins, minerals, and fiber, that are naturally occurring in healthy foods. They are health protectors for your body.

But since you cannot possibly obtain and consume every single nutrient your body and brain require through diet alone, you need to choose a good multivitamin. Look for "USP" on the label. This means that the product has been formulated to dissolve 75 percent after one hour in body fluids. In addition, look to see that the iron in the supplement is ferrous fumarate or ferrous sulfate, because they are the most absorbable forms.

Multivitamins always include vitamins C, D, E, K, and the Bs. Vitamin C maintains healthy gums, teeth, and blood vessels. Vitamin D aids in calcium absorption and the growth and strength of bones and teeth. Vitamin E protects cells from damage by free radicals. Vitamin K improves blood clotting. Vitamin B_1, or thiamine, is an antioxidant that enhances circulation and assists in the production of blood and hydrochloric acid. It also energizes you and promotes your learning capacity. Vitamin B_2, or riboflavin, aids in red blood cell formation. Vitamin B_3, or niacin (niacinamide, nicotinic acid), promotes healthy skin and good circulation. Vitamin B_5, or pantothenic acid, is called the antistress vitamin. Vitamin B_6, or pyridoxine, promotes cancer immunity and prevents arteriosclerosis by inhibiting homocysteine. Vitamin B_{12}, or cyanocobalamin, prevents anemia and helps your body to utilize iron.

Take your multivitamin with a meal instead of on an empty stomach; otherwise you may experience nausea. And make sure that your meal contains a little fat. The fat-soluble vitamins A, D, and E need a little fat to get inside your system and go to work.

Throughout this book, look for much more information about specific supplements.

BASIC BRAIN FOOD

Read the label on the supplement bottle, and understand what it means.

SUPPLEMENTAL BRAIN FOOD

You need to obtain many essential nutrients from supplements—your food will not provide enough.

FOOD FOR THOUGHT

BRAIN-BUSTING TIP-OFF #10: Don't neglect to take supplements because of the expense; consider it part of your nutritional budget.

BRAIN-BOOSTING TIP #10: Essential brain nutrients include the full range of vitamins and minerals.

SECTION 2

YOUR BRAIN AND YOUR MENTAL HEALTH

chapter 11

YOUR BRAIN'S LIMBIC SYSTEM

EEP WITHIN YOUR brain is a portion known as the limbic system. In the limbic system you will find the thalamus, amygdala, hypothalamus, and more. It is this system that deals primarily with behavior and emotions. This is the emotional storehouse of the brain, where motivating feelings such as anger, fear, and pleasure are born. The amygdala is the control area for two of the most complex functions of the brain, namely emotional responses and the processing of memories.

This linkage between memories and emotional response is important. For example, if you are walking down the street at night and you see movement in the bushes ahead, your "fight-or-flight" response starts up immediately. This could be something dangerous, and it's dark, so you can't quite tell. You hear the rustling of an animal, and you draw back with your eyes open wide. Then out comes the neighbor's little poodle, and you relax. Your memory of the harmlessness of the pet disarms your stress response, and you are able to call the pup over with a nice, "Here, Fifi!"

The limbic system is also responsible for regulating hunger, thirst, pain responses, aggressive behavior, and more. It will be the first part of your brain to pick up on the fact that it's time to eat, whether this is triggered by true hunger or an emotion-based craving.

Food cravings strike most people at one time or another, but if you find that you can't seem to resist that urge to raid the fridge after the late-night news or the snack machine in the break room at work, here are some healthy eating habits that can help to cut off unhealthy food cravings before they start.

1. Keep your blood sugar regulated by snacking on healthy, low-glycemic foods (cherries, grapes, strawberries, apples, carrots, peanuts, etc.) rather than waiting for your next meal. The less your blood sugar drops, the less likely you

will be to have a strong craving that you seemingly can't resist.

2. Eat a combination of carbs, protein, and healthy fat at every meal. Protein and fat take longer to digest than carbs do, so eating them with carbs and fiber means you'll feel full longer.

3. Purge your shelves of junk foods you tend to crave, such as cookies and chips, and replace them with bags of cut-up carrots and celery, low-fat cottage cheese, yogurt, dried fruits, nuts, and light popcorn.

4. If cravings strike when you're stressed, pausing to take a quick emotional inventory may help you discover the real reason behind your craving. Could a brisk walk relieve your stress instead of eating? Maybe a phone call to a friend to talk through a trying situation and pray about it together would provide more comfort in the long run than that tub of Ben & Jerry's.

BASIC BRAIN FOOD

Your limbic system is the source of emotions as well as a regulator of hunger and thirst.

SUPPLEMENTAL BRAIN FOOD

A phone call to a friend to talk through a trying situation and pray about it together would provide more comfort in the long run than that tub of Ben & Jerry's.

FOOD FOR THOUGHT

BRAIN-BUSTING TIP-OFF #11: Don't let cravings take over. Search inside to find the real reason behind your desire to eat.

BRAIN-BOOSTING TIP #11: Before your brain's limbic system detects your next hunger pang or craving, stock up on low-glycemic snack foods like grapes, strawberries, apples, and carrots to keep your blood sugar on an even keel.

chapter 12

ALL-IMPORTANT NEUROTRANSMITTERS

NEUROTRANSMITTERS, WHICH ARE important chemical messengers of the brain, help to control our feelings of anger, fear, anxiety, and depression. But when neurotransmitters are depleted, prolonged anxiety or trauma can overload the cerebral cortex of the brain, causing the release of adrenaline. When adrenaline floods the brain, it triggers a multitude of life-disrupting physical symptoms.

While emotions, especially panic and anxiety, involve the brain, they are also felt throughout the entire body because our brains control every cell in the body. Biological and possibly genetic factors may be involved when people experience crippling anxiety or other emotional illnesses. It also seems that a person's perception of traumatic events or stress can actually alter his or her brain chemistry.

Because fear, anxiety, and other dangerous emotions can alter the brain and body's chemical balance, they have a profound influence on the development of illness. In fact, prolonged stress can lead to eventual immune system breakdown. In other words, your emotions are not just "all in your head"—they are linked to the chemistry of your immune system.

Candace Pert, PhD, professor at the Center for Molecular and Behavioral Neuroscience at Rutgers University, made this statement in her research on the entire physiology of the body: "The chemical processes that mediate emotion occur not only within our brains, but also at many sites throughout the body, in fact, on the very surfaces of every single cell."[1] Early in Dr. Pert's career she discovered a way to measure chemical receptors on cell surfaces in the brain. At this particular time, Dr. Pert was studying opiate receptors in the brain, which act like keyholes for opiate drugs such as morphine. It is the binding of an opiate to its receptor that creates the emotion of euphoria.

Soon after, it was discovered that the body makes its own opiates called *endorphins*, which serve as natural painkillers. Our bodies release these endorphins or painkillers during events such as child-birth and traumatic injury. Later on, it was discovered that a host of other receptors besides opiates could be found in the brain, along with other natural chemicals called *neuropeptides*. However, not all neuro-peptides are associated with emotions as strong as euphoria. Some are more subtle, according to Dr. Pert. This groundbreaking information shocked the scientific community. The fact that endorphins were found in the immune system and that opiates and other receptors were found distributed in parts of the body outside the brain gave the mind/body connection credibility. This new research challenged the old notion that the immune system is independent of the nervous system.

Opiate receptors found in the brain were also found on immune cells. This opened the door and gave birth to mind/body medicine. Today, it is common knowledge among researchers and health-care professionals that the brain and immune system communicate with one another. Studies suggest that even very short bouts of dangerous emotions may alter some aspects of immune function.

This means that when dangerous emotions are not dealt with, or when an emotionally troubling situation becomes chronic or ines-capable, a person's immune system suffers and health problems arise. In other words, people who are under stress are more susceptible to illness.

Serotonin is a neurotransmitter that regulates your feelings of comfort, calmness, patience, and energy. When your serotonin levels are low, you may feel anxious, stressed, worried, angry, and fatigued. To increase your serotonin level, simply eat certain carbohydrates such as whole-grain breads or cereals, pasta, potatoes, popcorn, or rice. These cause your body to produce insulin, which allows tryptophan to enter your brain. Tryptophan is used by your body to create more of the neurotransmitter serotonin that will calm you down.[2]

The more we can learn about how our bodies react to emotional ups and downs, the better we can cooperate with health-producing prac-tices, including making good dietary decisions.

BASIC BRAIN FOOD

The foods you eat help manufacture neurotransmitters, the chemical messengers of the brain, which help to control our feelings of anger, fear, anxiety, and depression.

SUPPLEMENTAL BRAIN FOOD

If you are on medications to treat anxiety or stress, talk to your health-care professional about trying some natural stress busters instead.

FOOD FOR THOUGHT

BRAIN-BUSTING TIP-OFF #12: When you feel stressed, don't reach first for a drug.

BRAIN-BOOSTING TIP #12: When you feel stressed, take a popcorn break.

chapter 13

EMOTIONAL DISORDERS

As YOU WILL remember from chapter 11, your brain's limbic system is command central for all of the emotions you experience. When dangerous emotions are allowed to fester within us and we neglect to replenish our brains through proper nutrition and rest, full-blown emotional disorders can erupt. The following disorders have become commonplace. Each one of them is caused by brain, body, and spiritual depletion, and experts agree that life events, stress, grief, anger, and heredity affect the body's internal chemistry and contribute to their development.

- *Generalized anxiety disorder (GAD)* is characterized by excessive, nonspecific anxiety marked by excessive and unrealistic worries about health, money, or career prospects that last for six months or longer. People who live with GAD typically have a number of physical and emotional complaints, including insomnia, dizziness, concentration problems, sore muscles, restlessness, and irritability. Symptoms vary from person to person. GAD is often triggered by too much stress in the months or years immediately prior to its onset. (Note: Positive life events can also be stressful.)
- *Social anxiety disorder* is more than a case of just being shy. Social phobia is an anxiety disorder that tends to begin in the mid to late teen years and can grow worse over time. The central fear in this disorder is embarrassment over the way one might act while performing a task in public, such as public speaking, flying in a full plane, or riding in a bus or car. Symptoms include physical signs of nervousness such as trembling, blushing, and sweating.
- *Obsessive-compulsive disorder (OCD)* causes ritualistic, repetitive anxiety-relieving actions arising from a fear

of uncertainty and constant doubts. Some sufferers spend hours bathing, shampooing, washing their hands, or cleaning their homes. Many people with OCD also suffer from depression. OCD tends to run in families.

- *Post-traumatic stress disorder (PTSD)* is characterized by irritability; nightmares, insomnia and flashbacks; and "jumpiness," feeling the need to be constantly vigilant. PTSD results in brain depletion, and ongoing stress can make changes even in the structure of the brain. In addition, high blood pressure, cancer, and heart disease have been associated with this condition if it is left untreated. Called "combat fatigue" in the past, PTSD is now known to afflict anyone, male or female, who has suffered a traumatic event such as the unexpected death of a loved one, being assaulted, or being raped. Other triggers include auto accidents, a cancer diagnosis, miscarriage, and traumatic childbirth.

- *Panic disorder* symptoms vary from person to person and can include rapid or pounding heartbeat; sweating, trembling, or choking sensations; smothering or shortness of breath sensations; chest pain or discomfort; nausea, bloating, indigestion, or abdominal discomfort; dizziness, unsteadiness, light-headedness; feeling unreal or dreamy; fearing loss of control or going crazy; numbness or tingling sensations in the face, extremities, or body; chills or hot flushes; pallor of skin (or blushing or skin blotches); and the urgent need to urinate or defecate.[1] Also preceded by a traumatic or stressful event, this disorder appears to run in families and is two to three times more likely to strike women.

The four traditional forms of treatment include behavior therapy, medication, relaxation therapy, and cognitive therapy. Most people respond best to a combination of these options. In many of my books, I've shared a simple progressive muscle relaxation technique that I call MANTLE, which stands for **M**uscles **A**lways **N**eed **T**ension **L**oosening **E**very day. Simply tense and hold for the count of ten each part of your body, one section at a time, beginning with the muscles of your face and mouth, down through the other parts of your body: shoulders, arms, hands, fingers, upper abdomen, lower abdomen and pelvic area, upper thighs, calves, feet, and toes.

Another way to help manage stress and anxiety that lead to emotional disorders is through diet. Eliminate common food stressors like yeast, sugar, and dairy for a period of time and evaluate the difference in how you feel.

Food can affect your body's reaction to *stress*, and *stress* can affect your body's reaction to *food*. Food allergies and food intolerance can be exacerbated by stress and anxiety. If you have food allergies or food intolerance, eliminate these items from your diet if you have not already done so. Often, the body can tolerate these foods again if they are avoided for a time and then reintroduced to the diet slowly. If your allergic reaction to a certain food is severe, you should not try to reintroduce it into your diet without consulting a health-care professional.

BASIC BRAIN FOOD

The B vitamins aid recovery from anxiety disorders.

SUPPLEMENTAL BRAIN FOOD

For stress disorders, take GABA, magnesium, and the full spectrum of amino acids.

FOOD FOR THOUGHT

BRAIN-BUSTING TIP-OFF #13: Don't expect to resolve underlying emotional issues before the chemical balance of the brain has been restored.

BRAIN-BOOSTING TIP #13: To manage stress and anxiety that drain your brain, eliminate common food stressors such as yeast, sugar, and dairy.

chapter 14

FOR YOUR MOODS:
"DO" AND "DON'T" FOODS

THE FIFTH CENTURY B.C. Greek physician Hippocrates, now known as the Father of Medicine, is quoted as having said, "Let food be your medicine and medicine be your food."

Hippocrates knew what many of us are just finding out—that we can change our moods and our state of well-being through the foods we eat.

In Scandinavian and East Asian countries, where people tend to eat a lot more fish than we do in the United States, there tends to be a lower rate of depression. This is likely to be because of the additional omega-3 fats that the people obtain through eating fish; omega-3 fats are known to have antidepressant effects.[1]

Two scientists, Dr. Richard Wurtman and Judith Wurtman (Massachusetts Institute of Technology), were "the first to connect food with mood when they found that carbohydrate foods boosted a potent brain substance called serotonin."[2] I mentioned serotonin in chapter 12 of this book. Serotonin is a neurotransmitter, and when its levels are elevated, it helps you feel more calm and relaxed. It helps control not only your mood but also your ability to sleep, the quality of sleep you get, and your appetite. Author Charles Stuart Platkin writes about how serotonin works:

> The glucose in high-carbohydrate food triggers the release of insulin. This in turn allows the amino acid tryptophan to reach the brain (by blocking other competing amino acids), stimulating the production of serotonin.
>
> But when people feel down, they tend to go for foods that are not only high in carbohydrates, but are also high in processed sugar and fat. "When people are feeling gloomy, they attempt to self-medicate with food," says Elizabeth Somer, author of

Food & Mood. "They go to carbohydrates to feel better; unfortunately, they go to the wrong foods for the right reasons."[3]

To provide the right kind of food-boost for your mood, choose to:

DO	DON'T
• Drink more water • Eat more fresh fruits and vegetables • Eat more fish • Eat more "brown" (whole-grain) foods • Eat more protein • Eat more nuts and seeds • Eat more fiber and more organic food	• Consume large amounts of sugar • Drink caffeinated beverages • Drink alcohol • Consume large amounts of saturated fats • Consume foods that contain additives • Consume dairy and/or wheat products without caution[4]

BASIC BRAIN FOOD

Eat more fish to steer clear of depression.

SUPPLEMENTAL BRAIN FOOD

Supplement with amino acids, which are natural tranquilizers.

FOOD FOR THOUGHT

BRAIN-BUSTING TIP-OFF #14: Watch out for foods that contain additives.

BRAIN-BOOSTING TIP #14: You can improve your mood more by eating a piece of whole-grain toast than by eating a candy bar.

chapter 15

RECHARGING YOUR A BATTERIES

I

T'S COMMON TO feel "brain drain," or feel as if your batteries are dead when you have prolonged periods of stress or frequent emotional reactions such as anger, impatience, tears, or any emotion—even excitement. By now you know that stress affects your brain. Emotional fatigue is the manifestation of stress that you notice first.

It does drain your "batteries." Your adrenal glands are the two little glands that sit on top of each kidney. I call them your "A batteries." Your adrenal glands help your body deal with stress. They secrete adrenaline in crisis situations to give you the extra energy you need to handle an immediate crisis. They are part of your fight-or-flight response.

In days gone by, the fight-or-flight response was useful. It still is, once in a while, to get us out of the way of an oncoming automobile or the like. But when we get stuck in emergency mode because of our stressful lifestyles, our brains tell our adrenal glands to provide a steady stream of adrenaline, which was never intended.

Not only do our adrenal glands get exhausted, but we do too. Handicapped, our poor brains struggle to supply the right information at the right time. We make bad decisions, fall under the influence of rogue emotional responses, and generally do poorly. When our A batteries are drained, we feel sluggish and lethargic; our memories are dull; we get moody and touchy; we feel anxious, weak, and shaky. We may also suffer from hypoglycemia, low immunity, dry skin, brittle nails, sugar cravings, and profound fatigue.

If you want to see just how well your adrenal glands are performing, try this self-test. First, lie down and rest for five minutes. Then use a blood pressure monitor to take your blood pressure. Stand up immediately and take your blood pressure reading once more. If your blood pressure is lower after you stand up, you probably have reduced adrenal gland function, which means your batteries need a charge. The lower the blood pressure reading is from your resting blood pressure, the more severe your low adrenal function is. The systolic number (the number on top of the blood pressure reading) normally is about ten points higher when you are standing than when you lie down. A difference of more than ten points should be addressed.

Pay attention to your adrenal glands, your vital "A batteries," as you work to restore your system after a time of grief or conflict, prolonged pain syndromes, anxiety disorders, or depression.

To help support your brain and body during recovery from adrenal fatigue, eat meals that combine whole grains and proteins. Increase your veggie intake as well as your intake of oils such as olive oil, walnut oil, and fish oil. Avoid junk foods and caffeine, and don't skip meals, especially breakfast. Make sure to take a multivitamin daily.

Besides paying attention to your diet and vitamin intake, you might also decide to supplement with one of the following natural herbs, which have proven to help many people with the symptoms of stress:

- *Siberian ginseng*: a natural stimulant that improves oxygen and blood sugar metabolism as well as immune function. It's not advised for severe anxiety.
- *Valerian*: an herbal sedative widely used in Europe and China.
- *Passionflower*: an herbal remedy used for insomnia, anxiety, and irritability.
- *St. John's wort*: used for at least twenty-four hundred years to treat anxiety and depression. It enhances the activity of GABA and of three important neurotransmitters —serotonin, norepinephrine, and dopamine.
- *Kava*: a natural tranquilizer for both short-term and long-term treatment of anxiety, tension, fear, and insomnia. Kava acts on the brain's alarm center, the amygdala.
- *5-HTP (5-Hydroxytryptophan)*: related to the amino acid tryptophan. It is used to treat anxiety, insomnia, depression, and other related conditions linked with low levels of serotonin.
- *Vitamin C*: found in plants and especially fruits and leafy vegetables
- *Pantothenic acid*: also known as vitamin B_5

You can find more information about repairing stress damage in chapter 32 of this book.

BASIC BRAIN FOOD

Health-giving foods and naturally occurring supplements are your best choice for dealing with chronic emotional stress.

SUPPLEMENTAL BRAIN FOOD

Consider trying one of these herbal remedies: Siberian ginseng, valerian, passionflower, St. John's wort, kava, 5-HTP.

FOOD FOR THOUGHT

BRAIN-BUSTING TIP-OFF #15: If you are exhausted all of the time, even after a long night's sleep, it may be time to ask your doctor if you are suffering from adrenal fatigue.

BRAIN-BOOSTING TIP #15: Combine whole grains and proteins at meals to rid yourself of "brain drain" after a time of grief, conflict, prolonged pain, or depression.

chapter 16

DEPRESSION HAZE

A WELL-NOURISHED BRAIN IS more likely to be healthy and therefore able to keep your emotional state stable in spite of the stresses and difficulties of life. A person who is not depressed is more likely to eat a balanced diet, get adequate sleep, and undertake exercise, which further contributes to his or her good health.

While imbalances can lead to depression, depression itself often leads to changes in appetite, up or down. Increased appetite can result in unwanted weight gain, which in turn can lead to increased risk of high blood pressure, diabetes, and heart disease. Decreased appetite can cause weight loss and reduced intake of essential nutrients. Both can lead to fatigue and a lack of resistance to disease.

When you are angry, irritable, resentful, unforgiving, and uptight, your levels of the stress hormone called *cortisol* become elevated. Cortisol stimulates your appetite because one of its main roles in the stress response is to refuel you with carbohydrates and fats after you have completed the fight-or-flight response. Here's the catch, though. If you never complete the fight-or-flight response and leave your emotional stress-response motor running, the result will be an insatiable appetite for sweets—the quick fix for stress relief. This quick fix, unfortunately, leads to a quick expansion of your waistline.

Changes in food intake might mean reduced levels of some nutrients that have been specifically linked to depression, thus intensifying the problem. In particular, deficiencies in the B vitamins—folic acid, thiamin, riboflavin, niacin, and B_6—can lead to a clinical depression.

Signs of depression may include profound, persistent sadness and irritability; unexplained crying; low self-esteem; feelings of hopelessness, guilt, and emptiness; change in sleeping patterns or eating habits; restlessness; fatigue; difficulty making decisions, concentrating, or remembering things; a loss of interest in pleasurable activities, including sex; unexplained headaches, stomach upsets, or other physical problems that are not helped with standard treatment; and thoughts of suicide or death.

When certain nutrients are not supplied to our brains, a set of negative emotions can cascade and our ability to cope is compromised. But the answer is not just to take supplements, although they may help. If you follow a health-giving eating plan, you will begin to resupply your depleted brain and body with the nutrients they need.

When you are consuming a balanced diet, you will become more able to control your cravings because your cortisol levels will not be elevated. You will begin to be able to choose to snack on nutrient-dense foods that build your health without piling on the pounds.

Sometimes the smartest thing you can do for yourself is take a break, relax, and enjoy a high-protein shake. Your protein demands go up during stressful periods, and protein's building blocks, amino acids, are crucial for the health of your brain. If you are experiencing signs of depression, you should *avoid* alcohol, caffeine, and sugar, all of which cause changes in energy and mood.

BASIC BRAIN FOOD

Depression responds well to a high-protein, balanced diet.

SUPPLEMENTAL BRAIN FOOD

To get more protein, supplement your diet with the amino acids that you may be missing.

FOOD FOR THOUGHT

BRAIN-BUSTING TIP-OFF #16: Don't self-medicate depression with sugary foods or alcohol.

BRAIN-BOOSTING TIP #16: If you are feeling depressed, boost your mood and your brain function by enjoying a high-protein shake.

chapter 17

ADOLESCENCE, EATING DISORDERS, AND YOUR BRAIN

THE BRAIN IS hard at work as a teen transforms from childhood to adulthood. Adolescence is a time when the body undergoes many changes brought on by hormones, and the pituitary gland, a part of the brain's limbic system, is commander in chief of this transition.

Girls typically enter puberty around age twelve or thirteen, and boys at fourteen or fifteen. The physical changes during adolescence affect the body's nutritional needs, and healthy food choices are especially important during this time to support the growth of muscles and bones and to keep the brain functioning at its best.

Unfortunately, adolescence can also bring the onset of eating disorders (known specifically as anorexia nervosa, bulimia, and binge eating) as eating habits change and teens become more responsible for their own eating. Teens tend to be extremely focused on appearance and may feel peer pressure to look a certain way. Depression, anxiety disorders, and substance abuse often occur at the same time. Needless to say, when a person has an active eating disorder, he or she does not eat in a balanced, nutritionally sound manner, which only brings rational thinking and emotional reactions further into confusion.

The National Institute of Mental Health defines eating disorders as follows:

- *Anorexia nervosa*, in which you become too thin, but you don't eat enough because you think you are fat
- *Bulimia*, involving periods of overeating followed by purging, sometimes through self-induced vomiting or using laxatives
- *Binge eating*, which is out-of-control eating[1]

It is vitally important to get help for an eating disorder before it causes heart and kidney problems or even death. No one can overcome an eating disorder alone, and nutritional counseling is part of the solution. A person with an eating disorder can't just start eating normally. Far from being merely a food addiction (in the case of binge eating or bulimia) or a plea for attention, eating disorders are complicated behavioral disorders that involve a person's perception of himself or herself and the outside world as well as a self-aggravating downward spiral of health concerns.

According to the National Eating Disorders Association, "the most effective and long-lasting treatment for an eating disorder is some form of psychotherapy or counseling, coupled with careful attention to medical and nutritional needs. Ideally, this treatment should be tailored to the individual and will vary according to both the severity of the disorder and the patient's individual problems, needs, and strengths."[2]

Since the attitudes toward food and personal worth are developed early in life, a person's family of origin may be a place where nutritional counseling can be effectively coupled with psychological help. See chapter 16 ("Depression Haze") for more information about handling the depression component of eating disorders.

BASIC BRAIN FOOD

Treating the nutritional needs of an eating disorder may help balance the brain as psychological needs are addressed.

SUPPLEMENTAL BRAIN FOOD

Low levels of serotonin may be linked to eating disorders.

FOOD FOR THOUGHT

BRAIN-BUSTING TIP-OFF #17: Anyone suspected of having a problem with body image or with eating habits that match the descriptions of an eating disorder should seek the help of a counselor.

BRAIN-BOOSTING TIP #17: Watch for unhealthy changes in teenage eating habits, and reinforce the importance of proper nutrition for a healthy brain and body now and in the future.

chapter 18

TOO TIRED TO THINK STRAIGHT? MAYBE IT'S YOUR DIET.

I s YOUR BRAIN telling you you're too tired to keep going? There's a difference between being simply tired and being truly fatigued. When you're tired, it's temporary. After a relaxing weekend, you feel fine again. But when—day after day—you wake up in the morning so tired that you feel like your brain is in a cloud all day long, the idea of a nap suggests itself regularly, and you can't stop thinking, "I'm *so* tired," you are probably suffering from serious fatigue.

Address fatigue in practical ways. Are you making an effort to get enough sleep? Are you overcommitting yourself to activities and stretching yourself to the limit of your daily endurance? Perhaps you can make some changes in your lifestyle. In the meantime, and along with other changes in your life, how can you address fatigue nutritionally?

A frequent cause of fatigue is food allergies. Many people who complain of fatigue, depression, bloating, intestinal gas, nasal congestion, postnasal drip, and wheezing may suffer from a food sensitivity, also called food intolerance. Food allergies and sensitivities, especially the common intolerances to dairy products and wheat, can cause digestive disturbances and poor absorption of nutrients, which result in more fatigue. Ninety percent of food allergies and sensitivities involve the following foods: milk, eggs, peanuts, tree nuts (such as cashews and walnuts), fish, shellfish, soy, and wheat.[1] Experiment with your diet, or talk to your doctor about allergy testing to see if your problems with fatigue involve food allergies.

Dairy products are a prime suspect. Delayed reactions such as mood swings, dizziness, headaches, and joint pain can occur. Lactose is the predominant sugar in milk and cannot be digested by many people. Dairy substitutes that are full of calcium and are easy to assimilate include soy milk, rice milk, and almond milk. Try sorbet or other frozen desserts made from rice milk. Try soy, almond, or rice cheese. You may be able to watch all of your allergic symptoms disappear in about seven to fourteen days.

Another hidden cause of fatigue is iodine deficiency. A lack of iodine can impair your thyroid function, and a sluggish thyroid can leave you feeling tired and weak. You can do a self-test at home to check your iodine levels. Simply take a Q-tip, dip it into a 2 percent tincture of iodine (available at any drugstore or supermarket), and paint a two-inch square on your thigh or belly. This will leave a yellowish stain on your skin that should disappear in about twenty-four hours if your iodine levels are normal. If the stain disappears in *less* than twenty-four hours, that means your body is deficient in iodine and it has thirstily sucked it up. If that seems to be the case, keep reapplying the iodine every day at different sites on your body until the stain begins to last a full twenty-four hours. Not only will you have diagnosed your iodine deficiency, you will also have treated it! If you suspect poor thyroid function, you should ask your doctor to check your thyroid levels to determine whether or not you need to address the situation further.

Also take a look at your sugar intake. I go more in depth on this topic in chapter 40, "Shake Out the Sugar!" which you should read if you are dealing with any level of chronic fatigue. In chapter 26, I cover ways to help overcome chronic fatigue syndrome.

Always remember, the food that you eat is *fuel*. It should energize you, not sideline you with fatigue and bloating. To banish your fatigue for good, nutritional supplements may be required. Enzyme supplementation can help you assimilate your food more efficiently. You may find that both chronic allergies and chronic fatigue will disappear after you begin enzyme supplementation.

While is it possible to receive enzymes from raw foods that you eat such as mangoes, papayas, bananas, avocados, and pineapples, I strongly suggest that you make sure you are "enzymatically insured" by supplementing your body with digestive enzymes from a plant source. An ideal plant-based enzyme formula should contain protease (digests protein), amylase (digests starches), lipase (digests fats), lactase (digests milk sugar), cellulase (digests plant fiber), invertase (digests refined sugar), and phytase (breaks down phytic acid). The usual recommendation is to take two plant supplemental enzymes at the beginning of every meal.

Last but not least, be sure to stay well hydrated. Pure water will help all of your body's systems to work more efficiently. In addition, water will help transport nutrients for assimilation and help with proper elimination, removing fatigue-producing toxins in the process.

BASIC BRAIN FOOD

Perhaps your fatigue comes from hidden food allergies. Experiment with your diet to find out.

SUPPLEMENTAL BRAIN FOOD

Consider supplementing your diet with a plant-based enzyme formula.

FOOD FOR THOUGHT

BRAIN-BUSTING TIP-OFF #18: Banish table sugar!

BRAIN-BOOSTING TIP #18: Counteract "brain clouds" and fatigue by eating mangoes, papayas, bananas, avocados, and pineapples to get extra plant enzymes from your food.

chapter 19

WHAT DOES FOOD HAVE TO DO WITH IT?

THE LAST EIGHT chapters have all had to do with the connection between the food you eat and your mental and emotional health. As you can see, good nutrition has a lot to do with whether you are in your "right mind" or perhaps beginning to become confused and troubled. An anxious or depressed mind is an indicator of compromised mental well-being. Compromised mental well-being is, in turn, an indicator that a person's life is out of order, whether through his or her own fault or not.

We cannot control the genetic pool we came from or most of the circumstances that have formed us, but we can, to a large extent, control the food we put into our mouths. I am convinced that we can improve our mental and emotional health by eating wisely and nutritiously.

According to medical studies, there is abundant evidence that nourishment obtained from food has a direct impact on mood, cognitive function, and behavior. For example, in a Finnish study on the influence of nutrition on antisocial behavior of a large group of men who were incarcerated, it was found that "by comparing the number of their disciplinary offences before and during the supplementation, antisocial behavior was reduced by the supplementation of vitamins, minerals and essential fatty acids."[1] In another study, wintertime supplementation with vitamin D reportedly improved overall mood.[2] Study after study has shown the connection between nutrition and brain function. Some studies have shown that high omega-3 intake (primarily through a high-fish diet but secondarily through supplements) seems to lower depression. Folic acid deficiency, a stringent low-fat diet, and higher levels of dietary serine and lysine (amino acids) all seem to correlate with depression, as well as both cognitive and social functioning.[3] Conversely, as shown both by research and anecdotal experience, high protein intake increases mental sharpness.

It should be obvious by now that nutrition is important for all aspects of brain functioning. People whose diet is poor, either because of their economic status or because of poor choices, can expect to suffer from diminished mental performance, and it follows that the person will find it more difficult than ever to make better choices about nutrition. Supplementation may be the best solution, since, for instance, deficiencies of folate (folic acid), vitamin B_{12}, iron, zinc, and selenium tend to be more common among depressed people.[4]

It can be extra difficult to obtain so many depleted nutrients through food alone, even without the factor of diminished mental ability. But in any case, the link is a solid one—your nutrition definitely has a major effect on your mental health. In the long run—or even in the short run—you can't escape that fact.

BASIC BRAIN FOOD

Your nutrition has a major effect on your mental health, for better or for worse.

SUPPLEMENTAL BRAIN FOOD

Supplements may be the best way to supply depleted nutrients in times of mental distress.

FOOD FOR THOUGHT

BRAIN-BUSTING TIP-OFF #19: Eliminate bad food choices along with other harmful lifestyle habits.

BRAIN-BOOSTING TIP #19: Eating folate-rich leafy vegetables such as spinach can safeguard against depression, as well as improve cognitive functioning.

chapter 20

BAN CLUTTERED THINKING

S TRICTLY SPEAKING, "CLUTTERED thinking" doesn't have much to do with food. After all, one of the best remedies for clearer thinking is to increase oxygen to the brain, and food doesn't deliver oxygen to the brain; blood does. But it is my conviction that—especially when we're talking about our brains—the thoughts that we put into our minds are a form of nourishment. Therefore, we need to take a look at them.

As I have mentioned throughout this book, dangerous emotions can play a part in the development of disease. Your emotional life, controlled by your brain's limbic system, is the center or core of your life. It helps you express love and compassion. It also helps you feel hurt and pain. God intended for us to be emotional beings, not simply physical ones. Our emotions allow us to enjoy joyful, fulfilling, and heartfelt relationships with others. Our emotional self allows us to feel life from our core or heart.

Anger, anxiety, envy, sadness, and bitterness are dangerous emotions because they rob us of life. Dangerous emotions are like junk food. Just as a diet of sodas and potato chips can leave you without motivation and enthusiasm for life, so can a life without satisfying emotional bonding and happy experiences.

Such dangerous emotions and the intense thoughts that accompany them need to be balanced in the same way our nutritional intake does. It is not an impossible task. We *can* examine them and make good choices about them. In an important way, it doesn't matter how legitimate our grievances are. What matters is how we process things.

Will you nurse a grievance, or will you take the initiative to forgive? Will you choose to wallow in sadness, or will you seek to recover so that you can influence others for good? Take a hard look at your emotional "diet." What does the Bible tell you about these "nutrients"? Are they good for you? How can you stop chewing on them?

You may need to ask somebody to help you. After all, you have been living in this cluttered head of yours for a long time now. You're accustomed to it, although you don't really enjoy it. But it's difficult to decide what to do about it. You may need another person to help you de-clutter your cluttered mental and emotional thinking. Even if you don't have another person to talk with, you can start by praying. That's the best supplement in the world!

BASIC BRAIN FOOD

Dangerous emotions such as anger, anxiety, envy, sadness, and bitterness are like brain junk food.

SUPPLEMENTAL BRAIN FOOD

Prayer is the best supplement of all for your mental and emotional health.

FOOD FOR THOUGHT

BRAIN-BUSTING TIP-OFF #20: Just as a diet of sodas and potato chips can leave you without motivation and enthusiasm for life, so can a life without satisfying emotional bonding and happy experiences.

BRAIN-BOOSTING TIP #20: For clearer thinking, avoid high-fat foods that will raise cholesterol, clog arteries, and limit the flow of blood to the brain.

SECTION 3

YOUR BRAIN AND YOUR PHYSICAL HEALTH

chapter 21

MIGRAINES AND OTHER HEADACHES EATING YOU UP?

BECAUSE THE BRAIN is the control center of your body, any disease or unhealthy influence that it suffers can have far-reaching effects on the rest of your body, not to mention your ability to reason clearly and to remember things.

One of the most common brain-related complaints is the common headache, or, more seriously, migraine headaches. As most people know, a migraine headache can arise from various causes, including anxiety and stress, lack of food or sleep, exposure to bright light, or, in women, hormonal changes. The pain is often centered in a particular location, and it seems to pulse or throb. Sufferers become sensitive to light and sound, and they may become nauseated to the point of vomiting. Some people can tell when a migraine is about to start because they see flashing lights or have other visual disturbances.[1]

Nutritionally, what can you do about migraine headaches? Here is some basic advice, most of which involves avoiding potential headache trigger foods.[2] Even though some of these foods are considered brain boosters, avoid them if you suffer from migraines or other headaches. By trial and error, you can tailor your diet to your own situation.

FOODS TO AVOID

- Chocolate
- Cheese
- Monosodium glutamate (MSG)
- Foods containing the amino acid tyramine (found in red wine, aged cheese, smoked fish, chicken livers, figs, and some beans)
- Nuts, peanut butter
- Some fruits (such as avocados, bananas, and citrus fruits)
- Onions

- Dairy products
- Meats containing nitrates (bacon, hot dogs, salami, cured meats)
- Fermented or pickled foods

FOODS AND SUPPLEMENTS THAT MAY HELP

- Flaxseed, walnuts, and fish (omega-3 fatty acids)
- 5-hydroxytryptophan (5-HTP) supplements help raise serotonin levels in the brain, which may have a positive effect on sleep, mood, anxiety, aggression, appetite, and other migraine-triggering impulses.
- Magnesium, combined with the herb feverfew and vitamin B_2 (riboflavin), may help lessen symptoms for those who have infrequent headaches.

BASIC BRAIN FOOD

Experiment until you find out whether certain foods are triggering your migraines or other headaches.

SUPPLEMENTAL BRAIN FOOD

Try magnesium combined with the herb feverfew along with vitamin B_2 (riboflavin).

FOOD FOR THOUGHT

BRAIN-BUSTING TIP-OFF #21: Avoid specific migraine trigger foods.

BRAIN-BOOSTING TIP #21: Drinking more water may help alleviate the migraines some people experience when the brain begins to dehydrate.

chapter 22

STROKES AND TRANSIENT ISCHEMIC ATTACKS: THE NUTRITION LINK

S TROKES OCCUR IN two ways: when a blood clot blocks a blood vessel in the brain (ischemic stroke) or when a blood vessel ruptures and bleeds into the brain (hemorrhagic stroke). Both kinds of strokes constitute an emergency, and both require immediate medical attention.

What are the symptoms to watch out for? One or more of these will happen suddenly:

- Numbness or weakness of the face, arm, or leg (especially on one side of the body)
- Confusion, trouble speaking or understanding speech
- Trouble seeing with one or both eyes
- Trouble walking, dizziness, loss of balance or coordination
- Severe headache with no known cause

A transient ischemic attack (TIA) is a ministroke, with the same symptoms except that it comes quickly and goes quickly. It occurs when a blood clot briefly blocks a blood vessel anywhere in your brain. The symptoms usually disappear within an hour or a day at the most. TIAs can serve as a warning that a full-fledged stroke may occur, so people who have had TIAs should take precautions.

In the case of either a stroke or a TIA, it is important to go to the emergency room of your local hospital. Surgery may become necessary. In the meantime, practical steps can help, such as taking blood-thinning medicines, not smoking, getting exercise, eating a nutritious diet, and maintaining a healthy weight. It is important to address health issues such as diabetes, high blood pressure, high cholesterol, and heart or artery diseases.[1]

While no food or supplement can guarantee to prevent a stroke or cure its aftereffects, the following foods and supplements may help. Always consult your medical practitioner before making major changes to your diet or supplementation:

DO	DON'T
• Eat foods that have antioxidant properties such as blueberries, cherries, tomatoes, peppers, and squash. • Eat foods high in B vitamins and calcium, such as almonds, beans, whole grains (if no allergy), dark leafy greens (such as spinach and kale), and sea vegetables (seaweed). • Eat fewer red meats and more lean meats, cold-water fish, tofu, soy (if no allergy), or beans for protein. • Use healthy cooking oils, such as olive oil. • Ask your doctor if the following supplements might be helpful: alpha-lipoic acid, calcium, magnesium, omega-3 fatty acids, B_9 (folic acid), B_6, B_{12}, betaine, and antioxidant supplements such as vitamins C and E and beta-carotene.[2]	• Use trans-fatty acids found in commercially baked goods such as cookies, crackers, cakes, french fries, onion rings, doughnuts, processed foods, and margarine. • Consume coffee, alcohol, tobacco, or other stimulants.

According to a recent article in *USA Weekend*, the Framingham Heart Study reported that "eating three additional daily servings of fruits and vegetables reduced overall stroke rates by 22 percent and the risk of bleeding stroke by 51 percent."[3]

BASIC BRAIN FOOD

Taking care of your health is the best insurance against having a stroke.

SUPPLEMENTAL BRAIN FOOD

Taking antioxidant supplements may help to prevent cell damage from free radicals in your body.

FOOD FOR THOUGHT

BRAIN-BUSTING TIP-OFF #22: Take a kitchen inventory; get rid of products that contain trans-fatty acids.

BRAIN-BOOSTING TIP #22: Eating three additional servings of fruits and vegetables every day may reduce your risk of having a stroke.

chapter 23

INFLAMMATION AND NUTRITION

I NFLAMMATION CAN AFFECT almost every part of your body. Many times it is merely an inconvenience, but when it affects your brain, it's a serious problem. Meningitis (inflammation of the *meninges*, the membranes that encase your brain and your spinal cord) can sometimes occur in conjunction with encephalitis (inflammation of the brain itself). However, in this chapter, I will be giving you nutritional advice for dealing with inflammation anywhere in your body.

Inflammation is an important part of your body's immune response to infection, injury, or irritation. The redness of the inflammation you see on a skin wound comes from the extra blood that rushes to the area with its healing properties. You can't see it as well, but that's the same thing that happens when you have a sore throat or you overdo it when you play weekend football.

But inflammation often becomes chronic, and then it also becomes a problem. Perhaps it's the chronic pain of rheumatoid arthritis or the physical dysfunctions of lupus, multiple sclerosis, or psoriasis, all of which are autoimmune disorders (inflammation affecting normal body cells, as if the body is at war with itself). Research is starting to link many other conditions with inflammation, including heart disease.

Many attributes of our lifestyle, including high-sugar and high-fat diets and low levels of exercise, increase our tendency to experience unwelcome inflammation. Because inflammation is so pervasive, we should attempt any means at our disposal to keep it from taking over our bodies. To "dial down" your susceptibility to the unwelcome aspects of your body's inflammatory response, here are some nutritional suggestions:

TO OBTAIN ANTI-INFLAMMATORY OMEGA-3 FATTY ACIDS:

- Eat oily *fish*, and take *fish oil supplements* on the days you don't eat fish.

- Substitute *olive, walnut,* or *flaxseed* oil for safflower, sunflower, corn, sesame, and other polyunsaturated vegetable oils.

- Eat *walnuts, flaxseeds,* and *soy* foods.

FOR INFLAMMATION-FIGHTING ANTIOXIDANTS:

- Eat a wide variety of *fruits* and *vegetables,* especially *blueberries* and *kiwi fruit.*

- Take antioxidant supplements such as *resveratrol, grape seed extract, quercetin* (500–1,000 mg twice daily), *pycnogenol,* or *citrus bioflavonoids,* as well as *beta-carotene* (15 mg daily) and *vitamins C and E.*

Also:

- Use fresh *garlic, ginger,* and *turmeric* (curcumin), all natural anti-inflammatory agents.

- Include *sunflower seeds, eggs, wheat germ, herring, nuts,* or *zinc tablets* (15–30 mg daily) for zinc, which controls inflammation and promotes healing.

- Eat *pineapple* or take *bromelain* supplements (a digestive enzyme, 1,000–1,500 mg following a meal), which may help reduce inflammation.

- Try supplementing your diet with S-adenosylmethionine (SAMe), alpha-lipoic acid, and coenzyme Q_{10} (180 mg daily), which can act as inflammation fighters.[1]

BASIC BRAIN FOOD

You can take nutritional measures to prevent and control unwelcome inflammation in your body.

SUPPLEMENTAL BRAIN FOOD

Supplements such as S-adenosylmethionine, alpha-lipoic acid, and coenzyme Q_{10} may help reduce inflammation.

FOOD FOR THOUGHT

BRAIN-BUSTING TIP-OFF #23: Avoid safflower, sunflower, corn, sesame, and other polyunsaturated vegetable oils.

BRAIN-BOOSTING TIP #23: To lower inflammation throughout your body and brain, eat more blueberries and kiwi fruit.

chapter 24

SYNCOPE (FAINTING) AND WHAT YOU EAT

THE IMPORTANCE OF proper blood flow to the brain has been the underlying message of the last two chapters. I've explained that impaired blood flow to the brain can cause cloudy thinking and strokes. In this chapter, you will discover that it can also cause syncope, also known as fainting. The term *syncope* comes from the Latin and Greek words that mean "cutting short." Syncope or fainting is a temporary loss of consciousness due to insufficient blood flow to the brain.

When fainting is caused by an underlying health condition, that condition should be addressed first and foremost. At the same time, good nutrition plays a role in preventing fainting. In fact, the first piece of advice is the simplest—eat! As I am sure you know, the low blood sugar that results from not eating often enough can make you "feel faint." It is important to keep your body and brain fueled by eating modestly but regularly. Follow these commonsense guidelines for healthy eating:

- Eat plenty of fresh fruits and vegetables.
- Eat high-fiber foods, such as oats, fresh vegetables with peels, and beans. Take fiber in the form of psyllium seed supplements if necessary.
- Avoid refined foods (white breads, pastas, sugar).
- Choose fewer red meats and more lean meats, fish, tofu, and beans.
- Substitute olive, walnut, or flaxseed oil for polyunsaturated vegetable oils.
- Avoid trans-fatty acids, which are found in commercial baked goods (cookies, crackers, cakes, french fries, onion rings, doughnuts, margarine, and other processed foods).
- Avoid alcoholic beverages.
- Drink plenty of clean water daily.

- Get plenty of age-appropriate exercise at least several days a week.
- Supplement with fish oil capsules, a good daily multivitamin, coenzyme Q_{10}, acetyl-L-carnitine, alpha-lipoic acid, L-arginine, L-theanine, and adrenal hormonal extract if needed for adrenal stress.

In addition, if you have fainted more than once, try to determine the cause and avoid duplicating that situation. For instance, if heat makes you faint, avoid getting overheated. If you have low blood pressure and almost black out when you stand up too quickly, simply get in the habit of standing up carefully. Be more careful if you are taking a diuretic or any prescription medicine for which dizziness or faintness is a potential side effect.

BASIC BRAIN FOOD

What's the best way to keep from feeling faint? Eat!

SUPPLEMENTAL BRAIN FOOD

Supplement with fish oil capsules, a good daily multivitamin, coenzyme Q_{10}, acetyl-L-carnitine, alpha-lipoic acid, L-arginine, L-theanine, and adrenal hormonal extract if needed for adrenal stress.

FOOD FOR THOUGHT

BRAIN-BUSTING TIP-OFF #24: If you have trouble with fainting, avoid alcoholic beverages.

BRAIN-BOOSTING TIP #24: If you're feeling faint, eat fresh fruit or vegetables.

chapter 25

THYROID DYSFUNCTION AND YOUR DIET

Y OUR THYROID GLAND is located in the base of your neck on both sides of your lower larynx/upper trachea. The gland produces hormones to help control your body metabolism. Thyroid hormone is produced in response to another hormone secreted by your pituitary gland, which is right in the middle of your brain. In fact, your brain controls all of your thyroid's activity, so keeping your brain healthy through proper nutrition is the first step in normal thyroid function.

But sometimes the level of thyroid hormone can be too high or too low. The following symptoms accompany low thyroid hormone production, also known as hypothyroidism: fatigue, depression, weakness, weight gain, high cholesterol levels, low body temperature, and hair loss. When your thyroid hormone levels are restored, your energy level, weight, temperature, muscle strength, cholesterol, emotional health, and more will improve. If you can relate to any of these symptoms, see your health-care provider and ask for a thyroid health screening blood test, TSH (thyroid-stimulating hormone), free T4, and T3 tests.

Hyperthyroidism presents the opposite situation—an excess of thyroid hormone. Goiter (which is really an enlarged thyroid gland) may be present in both conditions.

There are natural supplements that can help correct thyroid dysfunction. Thyroxine is an amino acid that is excellent for people who have low thyroid function who also have prolonged, intense stress. L-tyrosine plays a crucial role in supporting the thyroid gland. Tyrosine boosts your metabolism as well as acts as the precursor for dopamine, norepinephrine, and epinephrine, which are nervous system chemicals that affect metabolism, mental alertness, and energy levels. Tyrosine can be taken in supplement form with a meal that contains protein. If your doctor finds that you are suffering from hypothyroidism, you may take L-tyrosine with your thyroid medication. Make sure to keep your thyroid monitored with periodic blood tests; you may be able to reduce or eliminate the need for medication.

Nutritionally, you will want to include the following foods in your diet in order to have enough iodine, which helps maintain proper thyroid function:

- Shrimp, lobster, oysters
- Seaweed
- Milk
- Iodized salt

If you have a low thyroid problem, you should steer clear of foods that interfere with thyroid function, such as broccoli, cabbage, brussels sprouts, cauliflower, kale, spinach, turnips, soybeans, mustard greens, peanuts, linseed, pine nuts, millet, and cassava. On the other hand, if you have an overactive thyroid, eat plenty of these foods. As usual, avoid refined foods, caffeine, and alcohol, and be careful of dairy and wheat-containing products.[1]

BASIC BRAIN FOOD

Your thyroid health is vital to your energy level and mental well-being.

SUPPLEMENTAL BRAIN FOOD

For low thyroid function, consider adding thyroxine and tyrosine.

FOOD FOR THOUGHT

BRAIN-BUSTING TIP-OFF #25: Foods that interfere with thyroid function include cruciferous vegetables, leafy green vegetables, soybeans, peanuts, linseed, pine nuts, millet, and cassava.

BRAIN-BOOSTING TIP #25: Iodine is needed for healthy brain and thyroid function; obtain it easily by using iodized salt, drinking milk, and eating shellfish and seaweed.

chapter 26

OVERCOMING CHRONIC
FATIGUE SYNDROME

C HRONIC FATIGUE SYNDROME (CFS) and Epstein-Barr virus are the result of lowered immune function and are accompanied by yeast infections, allergies, and virus activity. Many researchers believe that chronic fatigue syndrome is the result of a chronic infection with the Epstein-Barr virus, which is a latent virus that becomes active when normal immune response is compromised. The symptoms of this disorder include fatigue that does not resolve with bed rest, low-grade fever, throat infection, muscle weakness, gastrointestinal problems, sore lymph nodes, allergies, depression, loss of appetite, and weight loss.

This is an illness that I have experienced and have overcome. This disease is also related to hypoadrenalism or adrenal exhaustion. In addition, there is a strong connection to candida albicans yeast infection. This is clearly a stress virus that attacks the body when it is at its lowest point. It is a complex syndrome with a wealth of causative factors. The typical chronic fatigue sufferer is female, usually between thirty and fifty years old, outgoing, productive, independent, active, and an overachiever. This syndrome affects nearly two million people in America today. Considered medically incurable, it is increasing at an alarming rate. While it's true that no medical treatment or drug on the market today can help fatigue syndromes, and most hinder immune response and recovery, natural medicine offers hope and healing.

Charles W. Lapp, MD, cochairman of the Clinical Affairs Committee for the American Association for CFS and assistant consulting professor at Duke University Medical Center in Durham, North Carolina, says: "There is very little study of this aspect, but empirically my patients do best on a low-fat diet with lots of fresh fruits and vegetables, complex carbs (like rice and potato), and light meats (chicken, turkey, scaly fish)."[1] Lapp also says that people suffering with CFS are usually deficient in intracellular magnesium and vitamin B_{12}, whole body potassium, intracellular ATP, glutathione, taurine, serine, and the short-chain fatty acids such as valine, leucine, and isoleucine. He recommends supplementation with a multivitamin, magnesium, potassium, NADH, glutathione, and an amino acid capsule.

In addition to these health-building suggestions, I recommend that you read my book *90-Day Immune System Makeover* (Siloam, 2006). It will give you the plan that I used to regain my health, and it will truly help you rebuild and rebalance your entire body. This is crucial if you are going to overcome CFS. It takes about four weeks to realize improvement, and three to six months or longer to feel normal again. Most people do respond to natural therapies in three to six months. Many people achieve near normal functioning in two years time, even though the virus may persist in the body.

The following guidelines helped me and will also help your recovery.

1. First, you must strengthen your nervous system. I recommend a B-complex supplement, SAMe, boosting serotonin levels, or taking ginkgo biloba.

2. Boost your liver health with milk thistle seed extract and dandelion tea sweetened with the herbal supplement stevia. Apply warm castor oil packs to the liver area three times weekly.

Special considerations

- Aspirin, NSAIDS, or cortisone can hamper your body's ability to maintain bone strength and adrenal health.
- Avoid tobacco in all forms because it is an immunity destroyer.
- Have a protein shake each morning. This is crucial for rebuilding the body.
- Have a green drink (Kyo-Green from Wakunaga) for healthy blood chemistry.
- Symptoms are reduced by aerobic exercise. Begin with a short walk each day.
- Keep your bowel function optimal by adding fiber to your diet.
- Drink plenty of water, eight to ten glasses per day. This is especially important when increasing your fiber intake.

- Follow the eating plan as outlined in part 1 of this book.
- Limit sugar, caffeine, and alcohol.
- Use the herbal supplement stevia instead of sugar.
- Be patient with yourself. Recovery takes time. Be good to yourself; you deserve it!

BASIC BRAIN FOOD

Chronic fatigue syndrome cannot be cured with food, but good general nutrition is always helpful.

SUPPLEMENTAL BRAIN FOOD

Consider adding a B-complex supplement and protein shake to your nutritional regimen.

FOOD FOR THOUGHT

BRAIN-BUSTING TIP-OFF #26: Limit sugar, caffeine, tobacco, and alcohol.

BRAIN-BOOSTING TIP #26: To fight chronic fatigue and improve brain functioning, stay as active as possible, starting with a short walk each day, but not so much that you get fatigued.

chapter 27

FIGHTING OFF FIBROMYALGIA

U P TO TEN million Americans, mostly women, suffer from fibromyalgia. It's considered to be a stress-related immune disorder with the central cause being a low level of serotonin and reduced-growth hormone.

There's also a link between fibromyalgia and the brain. Research has shown that people with fibromyalgia have a lower flow of blood to the parts of the brain that perceive pain signals. They also have twice the normal level of a brain chemical known as substance P, which helps transmit pain messages from nerve cells to the brain.[1]

The causes of this pain are a compromised immune system often preceded by a stressful event, magnesium deficiency, or possible viral connection.

Symptoms include aching, musculoskeletal pain, fatigue, weakness, headaches, confusion, bowel problems, poor sleep, nervous symptoms, hypoglycemia, shortness of breath, and cardiovascular problems.

Although there is no known cure, symptoms of fibromyalgia may be greatly improved by the following natural therapies:

1. Avoid sugars, fats, red meat, and caffeine.

2. Take Kyolic garlic by Wakunaga daily.

3. Have a green drink daily.

4. Use royal jelly.

5. To reduce pain and inflammation, try:
   a. Balanced by Nature Glucosamine Cream
   b. Quercetin, 1,000 mg
   c. Bromelain, 1,500 mg

6. For brain balance, try:
   a. Brain Link (amino acid powder)
   b. Ginkgo biloba
   c. GABA

7. To assist the musculoskeletal system, try:
   a. L-carnitine, 1,000 mg
   b. Magnesium gelcaps and malic acid
   c. B-complex

8. Natural antidepressants to raise serotonin levels:
   a. SAMe, 800 mg daily
   b. St. John's wort, 300 mg daily

9. For restful sleep:
   a. Valerian root extract
   b. Kava kava
   c. Passionflower

10. To boost immunity:
    a. Vitamin C, 3,000 mg daily
    b. CoQ_{10}, 60 mg three times daily

BASIC BRAIN FOOD

Record your symptoms in a daily log. This information can help your doctor in setting up or adjusting your treatment plans.

SUPPLEMENTAL BRAIN FOOD

To better resist the symptoms of fibromyalgia, take supplements that strengthen your immune system and balance your brain.

FOOD FOR THOUGHT

BRAIN-BUSTING TIP-OFF #27: Talk to your doctor if you experience a combination of widespread pain for at least three months, fatigue, depression, muscle stiffness, and headaches.

BRAIN-BOOSTING TIP #27: Eating a low-fat diet with plenty of fruits, vegetables, and whole grains can help you manage fibromyalgia.[2]

chapter 28

CONQUERING CHRONIC PAIN

Chronic pain is physical pain, often unexplained, that lasts for a long time—weeks, months, or even years. Common symptoms include sharp, shooting twinges or a dull ache, numbness, muscle atrophy, and poor reflexes.

Chronic pain can be complicated because many times the source is unknown. The physical causes of pain usually include injury and illness, but chronic pain can also be caused by adrenal and pituitary exhaustion, obesity, internal or external tumors, poor nutrition, an overly acidic diet, and poor muscle development.

There are connections between the brain and chronic pain. The body chemistry that creates pain signals and sends them to the brain is affected by emotional and mental stress. Prolonged emotional and mental stress can eventually manifest as physical pain. Pain is almost always individual and signals us to attend to its underlying cause. Pain dampens your strength and spirit, causing depression. While painkillers allow you to temporarily ignore the pain so you can work, live, and function better, they do nothing to address the cause of the pain. In addition, pain relievers can be addictive or damaging to the stomach lining as well as the liver and kidneys.

Nutrition is a key factor in managing chronic pain. Your diet supplies your body and brain with the chemistry they need to make an inflammatory response. Inflammation can make your pain feel stronger and last longer, but making the following dietary changes can help balance your brain and body chemistry and, therefore, reduce your pain:

- Avoid starchy and sugary foods and any carbohydrates you don't need.
- Avoid artificial sweeteners, colorings, preservatives, hormones, antibiotics, and herbicide and pesticide residues in your food.
- Increase your intake of lean meats, fish, and eggs.
- Eat two or more cups of fresh vegetables daily.[1]

There are also natural methods to overcome pain in the body. They work at a very deep level in the body, relaxing, soothing, and calming the area in pain. The following recommendations have been proven to aid in the relief of many different pain syndromes.

- Consider chiropractic adjustments, massage therapy, and therapeutic baths.
- Consider magnet therapy.

Herbal pain relievers

- White willow bark—anti-inflammatory and analgesic
- Kava kava—relieves stress from chronic pain or injury
- Valerian—a sedative that will help you relax and sleep
- St. John's wort—for nerve damage and to lift the spirits

Use enzymes to reduce inflammation

- Enzymedica's Purify
- Bromelain
- Quercetin
- MSM
- Boswellia

Painkillers from nature

- DLPA, 1,000 mg daily
- GABA, 750 mg
- Glucosamine caps and Dr. Janet's Balanced by Nature Glucosamine Cream
- Magnesium, 800 mg at bedtime

BASIC BRAIN FOOD

Research suggests that losing as little as 10 percent of your current body weight can help decrease physical pain.

SUPPLEMENTAL BRAIN FOOD

Turn to enzymes to reduce inflammation and herbal pain killers to ease chronic pain.

FOOD FOR THOUGHT

Brain-Busting Tip-Off #28: Eating foods that leave your brain and body depleted of nutrients can increase your body's pain-producing chemistry.

Brain-Boosting Tip #28: Dietary changes can balance brain chemistry and reduce pain; start by eliminating starchy foods, sugars, artificial sweeteners, food colorings, and preservatives.

chapter 29

NOURISHING THE OVERTAXED BRAIN

WHILE WRITING MY book *Breaking the Grip of Dangerous Emotions*, I came across an interesting article titled "The Brain's Balancing Act" that was very informative. In essence the article said that working either the left or right side of your brain too hard can wreak havoc with your entire body. By stimulating the underused portion of your brain, balance can be restored. When your brain is in balance, your well-being increases, netting immediate health benefits.[1]

Let's examine this theory. The left side of our brain sees individual parts that make up a whole. It organizes, analyzes, and rationalizes information. It is also the verbal side of your brain, responding to speech and using words to name and describe things. It also keeps track of time and thinks in terms of consequences. The right brain addresses emotions and is affected by music, touch, and body language. It follows hunches and feelings rather than logic. It is the visual side of your brain responding to pictures, colors, and shapes. Overreliance on one side can create frustration and eventual brain burnout. As you have learned, what affects the brain also affects the body. So, the effects of brain burnout can lead to physical problems such as insomnia, headaches, and fatigue. This is because a body cannot be healthy if the brain is not in balance.[2]

Below is a chart developed by Ann McCombs, DO, who works with hemispericity. She has found that certain symptoms indicate a brain imbalance. Most symptoms are left- or right-side specific. There are, however, some signs that could indicate a strain of either side.

DON'T OVERTAX YOUR BRAIN

Signs that the right brain is overtaxed

- Staring off into space
- Feelings of panic

- Difficulty paying attention
- Feeling overly sensitive and emotional

For right brain relief

- Work on a crossword puzzle
- Organize your closet
- Play a game of logic (chess)
- Learn new software
- Develop a personal budget

Signs that the left brain is overtaxed

- Feelings of worry
- Difficulty communicating
- Inability to follow a schedule
- Difficulty problem solving

For left brain relief

- Dance
- Listen to music
- Cook or make a gourmet dish
- Play with your children
- Take a walk outdoors

By stimulating the underused side of your brain, balance occurs, and your brain drain goes right down the drain.

Another great way to enhance the health of your brain and other vital parts of your body is to supplement your body with lecithin. It has been said that lecithin does more to improve and preserve our health than any other nutrient.

Scientific studies show that we can repress or minimize age-related changes in our brain such as memory loss associated with aging through the long-term use of a lecithin supplement. This is very exciting for older persons and those who battle higher-than-normal cholesterol.

Lecithin is derived from soybeans and egg yolk. Food sources of lecithin include grains, legumes, fish, wheat germ, and brewer's yeast. Although these dietary sources of lecithin are readily available, it is difficult to eat enough of them to give you the amount of lecithin needed to be therapeutic and effective. That's why I recommend supplementation with lecithin granules. Two teaspoons daily may be added to food or juice.

You can also supplement with gingko biloba, known for its ability to improve memory, concentration, confusion, and dizziness. It is widely used in Europe to treat dementia. Gingko biloba comes as a capsule, tablet, liquid extract, or dried leaf for tea. Initial results may take four to six weeks, but you should see continued improvement after that time period passes.

BASIC BRAIN FOOD

You can boost your right brain with mental exercises such as crossword puzzles and sudoku puzzles, and your left brain with cooking or walking outdoors.

SUPPLEMENTAL BRAIN FOOD

Consider supplementing your diet with lecithin granules.

FOOD FOR THOUGHT

BRAIN-BUSTING TIP-OFF #29: Difficulties in concentration or communication could mean that one or the other sides of your brain are being overtaxed.

BRAIN-BOOSTING TIP #29: Enhance your brain health by eating sources of lecithin such as grains, legumes, fish, wheat germ, and brewer's yeast.

SECTION 4

REBUILDING YOUR BRAIN

chapter 30

WHAT HAS STRESS DONE
TO YOUR BRAIN?

To ONE DEGREE or another, all of us experience stress on a daily basis. Exactly what happens to you when you experience stress? The rate of your breathing increases to supply the necessary oxygen to your heart. Your heart rate increases to force more blood to your muscles and brain. Your liver dumps more stored glucose into your bloodstream to energize your body so that it can support an increased level of physical activity. You produce more sweat to eliminate toxic compounds produced by your body and to lower your body temperature. Stress worsens most disorders. Stress is a component in every disease, and improvement will be slower unless stress is addressed.

Stress builds up over time, and different types of stressors affect people in different ways. Long-term stress affects your brain, causing it to age prematurely and leaving it more vulnerable to damage from a stroke. The cortisol released by your body during stress can help you in a short-term situation, but prolonged raised cortisol levels have been shown to decrease the number of brain cells in the hippocampus, thereby affecting your memory.[1] What does your own body reveal about the level of stress you may be undergoing?

Low-level stress can manifest itself in subtle ways, such as short-temperedness, scowling or frowning, having "tired eyes," exhibiting a bored or nervous demeanor, or losing interest in activities that used to be enjoyable. If this level of stress is not addressed over time, another layer of stress gets added on top of it that includes increased fatigue, insomnia, overall sadness, outbursts of anger, fear, and even paranoia.

At that level of stress, underlying physical problems may begin to emerge such as chronic head and neck pain, high blood pressure, an upset stomach, and an overall aged appearance. People who are even more stressed develop frequent infections and illnesses, because stress can reduce a person's immunity. Stress-related ailments can include skin disorders, asthma, heart disease, kidney malfunction, and mental/emotional breakdown.

Learning to relax is one of the most crucial components of reducing the effects of stress. When you are highly stressed, your adrenal glands are in trouble, and you must address the lifestyle habits that are destroying them. Part of what this involves is eating healthy foods (which will mean eliminating caffeine and sugar), exercise, and getting enough sleep daily.

Your diet should contain seafood, brown rice, almonds, garlic, salmon, flounder, lentils, sunflower seeds, bran, brewer's yeast, avocados, and green "superfoods" such as Kyo-Green (available at your local health food store), which contain protein and all the B vitamins. An adrenal glandular supplement, which you can also find at your local health food store, will help to nourish and stimulate your exhausted adrenals. It will also help to reduce inflammation and increase body tone and endurance that is so often lost when we are depleted. When vitamins B and C are added or included in the adrenal glandular supplement, the results are even better. Candida, chronic fatigue syndrome, allergies, and blood sugar imbalances such as hypoglycemia and diabetes are greatly improved by taking an adrenal glandular supplement.

Your adrenal exhaustion may have been caused by unrelenting stress, or it may have come from long-term use of corticosteroid drugs for asthma, arthritis, or allergies. Too much sugar and caffeine in your diet or deficiencies of vitamins B and C can also contribute to adrenal exhaustion. Adrenal exhaustion is also common during the perimenopausal and menopausal stages of a woman's life. You may decide to try 2 teaspoons of royal jelly daily. This substance is the food of queen bees, and it is marketed in health food stores. It is rich in vitamins, minerals, enzymes, and hormones, and it possesses antibiotic and antibacterial properties as well as a high concentration of pantothenic acid.

It's worthwhile to learn how to de-stress your body and brain and learn how to keep yourself that way.

BASIC BRAIN FOOD

Are you deficient in vitamins B or C? Eat more foods rich in these vitamins.

SUPPLEMENTAL BRAIN FOOD

For help with stress, try adding a "green drink" to your diet, as well as an adrenal glandular supplement and royal jelly, all available at health food stores.

FOOD FOR THOUGHT

BRAIN-BUSTING TIP-OFF #30: If you are feeling stressed, don't let it keep you from eating nutritiously.

BRAIN-BOOSTING TIP #30: Arm your brain against the effects of long-term stress by eating more seafood, brown rice, almonds, garlic, salmon, flounder, lentils, sunflower seeds, bran, brewer's yeast, and avocados.

chapter 31

REPAIRING STRESS DAMAGE

I N THE LAST chapter, I discussed the negative effects that long-term stress can have on the brain. Now that you're aware of these dangers, you can see how "brain boosting" can sometimes be the same as "stress busting." Here are some powerful stress busters to help you create a foundation of good health while you boost your brain at the same time:

1. *Eat well.* Apply what you have learned in this book and from your own experience to gain the benefits of eating well. What is best for you? Besides choosing foods that are health producing, make meals a pleasant social time. Make menu planning, table setting, cooking, eating, and even dish washing enjoyable times with family and friends. Eating the right foods in the right quantities will keep you well enough to face distressing challenges.

2. *Sleep deeply* every night. Sound sleep is essential for maintaining your emotional health and a healthy immune system. Most people don't get enough sleep. Find out how much you need by sleeping without being awakened by an alarm clock for a period of time. When you awake naturally, don't you feel relaxed? If you have trouble falling asleep, establish a regular evening routine that does not include vigorous exercise or caffeine, adjusting your bedtime no more than an hour on weekends.

3. *Confide in a friend.* In times of stress, you need to be able to talk about your problems with someone who is concerned about you. It's important for you to be able to express yourself, to know that someone wants to hear about you. Laugh together too because laughter releases tension. Laugh about everyday things or watch a classic comedy together.

4. *Express yourself* in creative ways. Do you have a hobby? Indulge in it—painting, gardening, dancing, writing in a journal, refinishing furniture, playing a musical instrument, or singing with a group or when you're alone.

5. *Simplify* your life. Take inventory of how you spend your time, money, and energy, and decide whether you really want to continue doing all of those things. If you stop doing something, will you or your family suffer—or benefit? If you are over-extended, learn to use the magic word *no*. Find joy in the simple things; make time to stop and smell the roses.

6. *Exercise* your body. Regular exercise is a natural releaser of stress. Exercise enhances your mood. The increased circulation of your blood increases your general immune protection, and at the same time it helps to buffer the immunosuppression effect of stress. Exercise makes your body more fit for handling physical challenges. It doesn't have to be in a gym or structured in any way, unless that's what you prefer. You can work exercise into your daily life by taking the stairs instead of the elevator, parking farther from your destination and walking to it, or tossing a ball in the backyard with your child or your dog.

7. *Make time to unwind.* It's all right to do "nothing." You could set aside a period of time every day to relax and listen to music. You could take a warm bath. You could take a stroll around the neighborhood or find a comfortable place to practice deep breathing. You could use aromatherapy (choose lavender, sandalwood, clary sage, lemon, neroli [orange blossom], or bergamot). Whatever you choose, make sure it's an activity that makes you feel refreshed, renewed, and rejuvenated.

8. *Give of yourself.* Helping someone else is one of the best ways to get your mind off your own problems. But if you feel extra-stressed, just use the time to *pamper yourself.* (Just be sure to pamper yourself in a health-producing way. Eating a pint of Häagen-Dazs does not qualify!)

9. *Keep a clear head* at all times. Alcohol or drugs will not cure stress. Your immune system is already suppressed

by your stress—you don't need to suppress it any more by using drugs or ingesting alcohol.

10. Try one of these stress-busting herbs: *Siberian ginseng* (helps your body to adapt to stress and reduces fatigue, although it is a stimulant, therefore not advised for severe anxiety or if you have high blood pressure), valerian (a natural sedative that enhances the activity of GABA), passionflower (often combined with valerian as an herbal remedy for insomnia, anxiety, and irritability), St. John's wort (used to treat anxiety and depression, enhancing the activity of GABA as well as the activity of three important neurotransmitters—serotonin, norepinephrine, and dopamine), kava (a natural tranquilizer that can help with anxiety, tension, fear, and insomnia), or 5-HTP (5-Hydroxytryptophan, which is related to the amino acid tryptophan, used to treat anxiety, insomnia, depression, and other related conditions linked with low levels of serotonin).

BASIC BRAIN FOOD

Dial down your stress level—it really is all right to "do nothing" sometimes!

SUPPLEMENTAL BRAIN FOOD

Stress-busting herbal supplements include Siberian ginseng, valerian, passionflower, St. John's wort, kava, and 5-HTP.

FOOD FOR THOUGHT

BRAIN-BUSTING TIP-OFF #31: Alcohol or drugs will not cure stress.

BRAIN-BOOSTING TIP #31: Eating the right foods in the right quantities—preferably in the pleasant company of other people—will relieve stress and equip your brain to face distressing challenges.

chapter 32

UNDOING PSYCHOSOMATIC KNOTS

I T IS IMPORTANT to recognize the unseen connection between our thinking and our bodies. The connection seems to be more obvious with certain disorders, such as colitis, migraine headaches (or even so-called "tension headaches"), immune disorders, and heart disease. Some of the connections involve stress, which we just discussed in the previous two chapters, and stress touches many body functions, such as blood pressure and the manufacturing of stomach acids. It seems likely that almost any physical disorder has a psychological component.

The study of this mind-body connection is called psychophysiology or simply "mind-body medicine." A cultural shift has been taking place in the United States and other Western countries for some time, so that the integration of mind and body is no longer considered to be an unusual concept. Increasingly, psychological and complementary models of treatment can coexist with traditional treatment of physical symptoms of disease. This means that the study of personal food and food supplement choices and the benefits that can arise from generally improved nutrition can fit better than ever into the discussion of attaining and maintaining maximum health.

One of the biggest advantages of undertaking changes in one's diet is that it carries a fairly low risk to do so. You can try a new food or drop a food out of your diet to see if your physical condition and your outlook seem to be affected by it. You can choose to increase your consumption of a whole class of foods, such as the foods that contain omega-3 fatty acids. You can begin to monitor your overall intake of calories and the foods that you tend to choose, to see if you may be sabotaging your health in some way. Since low blood sugar can affect the way you think and feel, it can sometimes enhance psychosomatic conditions. Snacking on healthy, low-carb foods between meals and combining proteins and carbs at all meals and snacks can help to keep blood sugar levels from dipping. Ongoing research into the mind-body connections and into nutrition will likely enhance our ability to make such decisions. Our health and quality of life cannot help but improve, even if we continue to live with a chronic condition or an inherited weakness.

Because mind-body medicine focuses on the interconnectedness of the brain, mind, body, and behavior, it "regards as fundamental an approach that respects and enhances each person's capacity for self-knowledge and self-care, and it emphasizes techniques that are grounded in this approach."[1] For this reason it is easy to see how nutritional considerations fit into the picture. Each person, always learning about his or her own body, can apply nutritional wisdom to health issues that link both brain and body, helping to bring improved mental as well as physical health.

BASIC BRAIN FOOD

Your mind and your body communicate with each other, for better or for worse.

SUPPLEMENTAL BRAIN FOOD

Learn all you can about your personal nutritional sufficiencies and deficiencies so you can maintain and improve your health.

FOOD FOR THOUGHT

BRAIN-BUSTING TIP-OFF #32: Don't let your brain ignore the signals that your body is giving it.

BRAIN-BOOSTING TIP #32: Snacking on low-carb foods between meals can help to keep blood sugar levels from dipping and affecting your brain-body connection.

chapter 33

THINKING THROUGH TO HEALTH: RECOVERY FROM A MAJOR ILLNESS

EATING THE RIGHT foods for your brain's health can also help your body fight off major illnesses and disease. When you are recovering from a major illness, what specific guidelines can you follow?

Cancer is one of the most prevalent major illnesses in the United States—and one of the most feared. Food-related approaches to recovery from this major disease include fasting—not eating at all or eating/drinking from a very limited menu. Other nutritional approaches to preventing or recovering from cancer include a diet of the following:

- Broccoli
- Garlic or garlic supplements
- Grapes or supplements of grape extract (for proanthocy-anidins) and grape skins (for resveratrol)
- Fruit and vegetable juice
- Fresh tomatoes (for lycopene)
- Fish or supplements for omega-3 fatty acids
- Apples, onions, teas, or quercetin supplements
- Sea vegetables (such as seaweed) or supplements
- Soybeans in various forms
- Vegetables only (no meat)
- Wheatgrass ("green drinks")[1]

Drinking at least one pint of juice each day is also helpful in the case of other major disorders. Fruit juices are the cleansers of our bodies, and vegetable juices are the builders and regenerators of our systems. Vegetable juices contain all the minerals, salts, amino acids, enzymes, and vitamins that the human body requires. Juices are digested and assimilated within ten to fifteen minutes after consumption, and they are used almost completely by your body to nourish and regenerate your cells, tissues, glands, and organs. The end result is very positive. Choose one of more from these combinations recommended for various conditions:

- *Arthritis*: celery, grapefruit, carrot and spinach, carrot and celery
- *Gallstones*: carrot and beet and cucumber, carrot and spinach, carrot and celery and parsley
- *Ulcers*: cabbage, carrot and spinach, carrot and beet and cucumber
- *Liver problems*: carrot, carrot and beet and cucumber, carrot and spinach
- *Bronchitis*: carrot and spinach, carrot and dandelion, carrot and beet and cucumber

Nutritional approaches cannot claim to cure a major disease such as cancer. But they certainly may help provide all-important nutrients at a time when they are needed more than ever.

BASIC BRAIN FOOD

Take charge of your recovery by taking charge of your nutrition.

SUPPLEMENTAL BRAIN FOOD

For lists of nutrient values of specific foods, see the 2005 Dietary Guidelines for Americans at http://www.health.gov/dietaryguidelines/dga2005/document/default.htm.

FOOD FOR THOUGHT

BRAIN-BUSTING TIP-OFF #33: When you are sick, don't leave your nutrition out of your recovery equation.

BRAIN-BOOSTING TIP #33: Consider juicing certain health-promoting fruits and vegetables to get the nutrients you need to boost your brain as you recover from illness.

chapter 34

REPAIRING DAMAGE FROM DRUGS OR ALCOHOL

THROUGHOUT THIS BOOK I have recommended that as a part of their good nutritional habits, people should abstain from alcohol consumption. But what if it's too late? What if a person has already inflicted significant damage on his or her brain through the excessive drinking of alcohol (or abuse of drugs, which can have equally negative effects on the brain)? Can good nutrition help to reverse some of the brain damage? This question is addressed by the following summary from the National Institute on Alcohol Abuse and Alcoholism:

> Alcoholics often eat poorly, limiting their supply of essential nutrients and affecting both energy supply and function maintenance. Furthermore, alcohol interferes with the nutritional process by affecting digestion, storage, utilization, and excretion of nutrients.[1]
>
> ... Alcohol inhibits the breakdown of nutrients into usable molecules by decreasing secretion of digestive enzymes from the pancreas.[2] Alcohol impairs nutrient absorption by damaging the cells lining the stomach and intestines and disabling transport of some nutrients into the blood....
>
> Even if nutrients are digested and absorbed, alcohol can prevent them from being fully utilized by altering their transport, storage, and excretion. Decreased liver stores of vitamins such as vitamin A, and increased excretion of nutrients such as fat, indicate impaired utilization of nutrients by alcoholics.
>
> The three basic nutritional components found in food—carbohydrates, proteins, and fats—are used as energy after being converted to simpler products. Some alcoholics ingest as much as 50 percent of their total daily calories from alcohol, often neglecting important foods.[3]

...Because cells are made mostly of protein, an adequate protein diet is important for maintaining cell structure, especially if cells are being damaged. Research indicates that alcohol affects protein nutrition by causing impaired digestion of proteins to amino acids, impaired processing of amino acids by the small intestine and liver, impaired synthesis of proteins from amino acids, and impaired protein secretion by the liver.[4]

Nutrients are essential for proper body function; proteins, vitamins, and minerals provide the tools that the body needs to perform properly. Alcohol can disrupt body function by causing nutrient deficiencies and by usurping the machinery needed to metabolize nutrients. Vitamins are essential to maintaining growth and normal metabolism because they regulate many physiological processes. Chronic heavy drinking is associated with deficiencies in many vitamins because of decreased food ingestion and, in some cases, impaired absorption, metabolism, and utilization.[5] For example, alcohol inhibits fat absorption and thereby impairs absorption of the vitamins A, E, and D that are normally absorbed along with dietary fats....[6]

Vitamins A, C, D, E, K, and the B vitamins, also deficient in some alcoholics, are all involved in wound healing and cell maintenance.[7] In particular, because vitamin K is necessary for blood clotting, deficiencies of that vitamin can cause delayed clotting and result in excess bleeding. Deficiencies of other vitamins involved in brain function can cause severe neurological damage.

Deficiencies of minerals such as calcium, magnesium, iron, and zinc are common in alcoholics....Deficiencies seem to occur secondary to other alcohol-related problems: decreased calcium absorption due to fat malabsorption; magnesium deficiency due to decreased intake, increased urinary excretion, vomiting, and diarrhea;[8] iron deficiency related to gastrointestinal bleeding;[9] and zinc malabsorption or losses related to other nutrient deficiencies....[10]

Nutritional deficiencies can have severe and permanent effects on brain function....Because alcoholics tend to eat poorly—often eating less than the amounts of food necessary to provide sufficient carbohydrates, protein, fat, vitamins A and C, the B vitamins, and minerals such as calcium and iron—a major concern is that alcohol's effects on the digestion of food and utilization of nutrients may shift a mildly malnourished person toward severe malnutrition.

The combination of an adequate diet and abstention from alcohol is the best way to treat malnourished alcoholic patients. Nutritional supplements have been used to replace nutrients deficient in malnourished alcoholics in an attempt to improve their overall health.[11]

In a similar vein, the director of the National Institute on Drug Abuse has testified that, regarding the abuse of drugs such as Ecstasy, methamphetamines, and others, brain damage and other physical damage is inevitable:

3,4-methylenedioxymethamphetamine, which is commonly abbreviated and referred to as MDMA or "Ecstasy," is an illegal drug that has characteristics of both stimulants and hallucinogens....It enables users to dance for extended periods, which can lead to hyperthermia, dehydration, hypertension, and heart or kidney failure....

MDMA works in the brain by increasing the activity levels of at least three neurotransmitters: serotonin, dopamine, and norepinephrine. Much like the way amphetamines work, MDMA causes these neurotransmitters to be released from their storage sites in neurons resulting in increased brain activity. Compared to the very potent stimulant, methamphetamine, MDMA causes greater serotonin release and somewhat lesser dopamine release....By releasing large amounts of serotonin and also interfering with its synthesis, MDMA causes the brain to become significantly depleted of this important neurotransmitter. As a result, it takes the human brain time to rebuild its serotonin levels. For people who take MDMA at moderate to high doses, depletion of serotonin may be long-term....

In short, there is now a large body of evidence that links heavy and prolonged MDMA use to confusion, depression, sleep problems, persistent elevation of anxiety, aggressive and impulsive behavior and selective impairment of some working memory and attention processes.[12]

As a result of this kind of research and testimony, you can assume that when brain damage has occurred as a result of the abuse of either alcohol or drugs, recovery can be improved through nutritional avenues.

BASIC BRAIN FOOD

Take measures to improve overall food absorption.

SUPPLEMENTAL BRAIN FOOD

Restore lost vitamins as part of nutritional therapy for damage from alcohol or drugs.

FOOD FOR THOUGHT

BRAIN-BUSTING TIP-OFF #34: Don't drink alcohol! Don't take drugs!

BRAIN-BOOSTING TIP #34: Basic good nutrition improves recovery from brain damage that has resulted from the abuse of alcohol or drugs.

chapter 35

GETTING YOUR FEET ON THE GROUND

I f you're feeling light-headed, it may be time for a quick brain-boosting food solution, but first you need to determine the cause. Light-headedness, or dizziness, and vertigo are two complaints that occur in conjunction with many disorders. Dizziness and vertigo do differ from each other, although they're hard to differentiate. Vertigo is usually defined as feeling that the room is spinning, and dizziness is usually described as feeling that your head is spinning. Either way, you are unstable on your feet and you feel light-headed. With vertigo, you might feel nauseated, even to the point of vomiting, and you can have ringing in your ears.

An inner ear disorder is often at the root of vertigo. Sometimes you will have tinnitus (ringing in one or both ears). If you are dizzy often, be sure to see your health-care provider to determine the cause.

Ringing in the ears and dizziness can also be symptoms of hypertension (high blood pressure), which can be caused by too much sodium (salt) in your diet. To help prevent high blood pressure, make sure you're getting plenty of magnesium in your diet, besides cutting back on salt. Dietary sources for magnesium include dairy products, meats, fish, nuts, molasses, brewer's yeast, avocados, and bananas.

With all the awareness people have these days about the dangers of high blood pressure, it might seem as if low blood pressure is a good thing to strive for. But lower is not always better. Severe low blood pressure can rob your brain of oxygen. This is what creates the light-headedness or dizziness that can accompany this condition.

If your blood pressure is continually 100/60 or below, you have low blood pressure. With it come fatigue, low energy, light-headedness when standing up, nervousness, allergies, and low immunity. The causes for low blood pressure include endocrine or nerve disorders, reaction to medications, electrolyte loss (for instance, from sweating heavily), weak adrenal function, and emotional distress.

Salt is one of your body's most important minerals, along with potassium and magnesium. Salt helps regulate the water balance of your cells. People with low blood pressure or low adrenal function can benefit greatly by adding ⅛ teaspoon of sea salt to an 8-ounce glass of spring water every morning to help increase blood volume and adrenal function.

Most people, however, consume too much salt. Do you get enough salt—or too much? It is very easy to do these days due in part to our fast-paced lives in which we dine out or buy frozen dinners frequently, or habitually oversalt our foods by salting them when we're cooking and again when we sit down to eat.

Dizziness can also result from something as simple as dehydration, which can also give you headaches and make you feel fatigued. Remember to drink plenty of clean, fresh water every day, all day long.

BASIC BRAIN FOOD

Dietary sources for magnesium include dairy products, meats, fish, nuts, molasses, brewer's yeast, avocados, and bananas.

SUPPLEMENTAL BRAIN FOOD

Be sure you're getting enough salt and other minerals in your diet.

FOOD FOR THOUGHT

BRAIN-BUSTING TIP-OFF #35: Check your salt intake. Too much salt can contribute to high blood pressure and not enough can open the door to low blood pressure.

BRAIN-BOOSTING TIP #35: If you feel light-headed and dizzy, you might be dehydrated. Boost your brain and get rid of dizziness by drinking more water.

chapter 36

SLEEPING IT OFF

YOU KNOW YOU need to get enough sleep, because lack of sleep can impair your brain's performance almost as much as a lack of oxygen or water. But it's too easy to eat or drink something that produces wakefulness instead of sleep. Foods and beverages to avoid before bedtime include anything that stimulates the neurochemical reactions in your brain, thus perking you up and sharpening your attention—and causing insomnia.

The primary stimulant you should avoid before bedtime is caffeine (especially coffee, tea, and colas). You may need to cut back on your caffeine intake during the earlier part of the day as well. You should be aware that over-the-counter cold and headache remedies may contain caffeine.

Alcohol is another stimulant you should avoid. A glass of wine may make you feel relaxed and sleepy before you go to bed, but as your body processes it, the sedative properties give way to arousing ones. This tends to jolt you awake during REM (rapid eye moment) sleep, just when you need to stay asleep.

Never eat heavy foods at bedtime, especially if they are sugary or spicy. Large meals make your digestive system work too hard, just when you want to settle down for the night. In particular, avoid meals close to bedtime that include chocolate, ham, bacon, sauerkraut, sausage, cheese, eggplant, spinach, tomatoes, sugar, and wine. These foods contain tyramine. Tyramine encourages the release of norepinephrine, which is a brain stimulant. You may also be sensitive to additives, preservatives, or agents such as MSG (monosodium glutamate).

Large or rich snacks will have the same effect as a large meal. In general, be kind to your digestive system—respect the fact that it will be moving more slowly at night. If you eat a high-protein snack (such as meat) before bedtime, you may feel too alert to go to sleep. Protein inhibits sleep by blocking the synthesis of serotonin.

To avoid having to interrupt your sleep to urinate, limit your fluid intake in the evening hours before bedtime. It's true that you need plenty of water during your day, and it's also true that you will sleep better if you are well hydrated in general. Just try to drink most of your water earlier in the day. If you aren't concerned about evening fluid intake, a warm cup of golden chamomile tea might be a perfect sleep-inducer. It has a mildly sedating effect, and, of course, brewing it and sipping it will provide you with a built-in time of relaxation before bedtime. Use 2 or 3 heaping teaspoons of flowers per cup of boiling water and let it steep five to ten minutes.

What foods will help promote restful sleep? Milk—especially warm milk—is the traditional bedtime sleep inducer because it contains tryptophan, an amino acid that, when converted to seratonin and melatonin in the body, makes you sleepy and helps to keep you from waking up in the night. These neurotransmitters tell your nerves to slow down so your brain can slow down too. Milk also contains calcium, which will help your brain to use the tryptophan. Some people swear by a little honey in their warm milk. Sugar in large quantities will have the opposite effect, but a touch of glucose causes your brain to turn off a neurotransmitter called *orexin* that helps to keep you alert and awake. The tryptophan and calcium are not affected by warming, so you can gain the same benefits from cold milk.

To get your brain even more calmed down, combine complex carbohydrates with milk or another tryptophan-containing food. What you don't want to do is eat a lot of protein *without* carbohydrates, because protein-rich foods contain the amino acid tyrosine, which will perk your brain up. Your best choice for a bedtime snack would include both complex carbohydrates and protein, along with some calcium. Eat high-protein, lower-carbohydrate meals for breakfast and lunch when you need to be at your best mentally. Then eat your dinner early enough so that it can digest before you go to bed.

Meals that are high in complex carbohydrates and low to medium in protein will help you relax during the evening and make a good night's sleep easy to achieve. Eat modestly so you are not overstuffed, but be sure to eat enough so that you won't get so hungry that you eat too much for a bedtime snack. If you do need or want a bedtime snack, eat it an hour or two before you turn in for the night to give the tryptophan time to work on your behalf. An evening snack that is high in junk sugars is much less likely to help you sleep. Besides missing out on tryptophan, you may cause your blood sugar to spike, then plummet, followed by the release of stress hormones that will keep you awake.

You might decide to try a sleep-inducing supplement. Amino acids such as 5-HTP (5-Hydroxytryptophan) acts as a precursor to tryptophan, which stimulates serotonin production in your brain to help to alleviate anxiety. Herbs such as kava, passionflower, and valerian have been used across the world for centuries for their natural sedative qualities. Calcium and magnesium, while available in some of the suggested sleep-inducing foods such as milk and bananas, are easy to obtain in supplement form. Inositol can ensure that you will not suffer from disturbed REM (rapid eye movement) sleep.

I tell my clients to avoid over-the-counter sleeping pills because of their undesirable consequences, which include lack of REM sleep (your dreaming sleep, which is essential), "hangovers," and a tendency to decrease in their effectiveness with overuse because of increased tolerance.

BASIC BRAIN FOOD

To encourage good sleep, avoid stimulants and choose foods that are rich in tryptophan and calcium.

SUPPLEMENTAL BRAIN FOOD

Natural sleep-inducing supplements include 5-HTP, kava, passionflower, valerian, calcium, magnesium, and inositol.

FOOD FOR THOUGHT

BRAIN-BUSTING TIP-OFF #36: Avoid heavy dinners and large bedtime snacks.

BRAIN-BOOSTING TIP #36: Warm milk induces sleep and helps your brain slow down to be rejuvenated while you rest.

chapter 37

SMART WEIGHT MANAGEMENT: GOOD FOR YOUR BRAIN TOO

O BESITY LEADS TO high blood pressure, which lowers cognitive function. Being overweight can also trigger depression, which leads to slower thinking. If you're overweight, a key to boosting your brain may be weight loss. Even moderate weight loss can change your body chemistry for the better, lower your blood pressure, and boost your brain.

The key thing to remember about maintenance of weight loss is balance. Don't starve yourself for days only to gorge yourself in response. Don't skip meals. It's best to eat several small meals daily instead of skipping meals and eating one big meal daily. You want to give your body even-burning fuel throughout the day. Otherwise, your body will store fat for survival instead of burning it. Make sure each meal and snack contains carbohydrates to provide glucose for your brain, protein for building and repairing muscles and releasing glucagon (your fat-burning hormone), and fat to supply fatty acids needed for blood sugar control, appetite suppression, and hormone production.

I recommend the following dietary guidelines to help you choose the foods that can most help you achieve balance in your weight. A high-fiber diet is necessary, because fiber improves the excretion of fat, improves glucose tolerance, and gives you a feeling of fullness and satisfaction.

Emphasize the following foods: brown rice, tuna, chicken, white fish, fresh fruits and vegetables, high-protein lean foods, lentils, beans, whole-grain breads, and turkey. Add healthy fats to your diet, such as olive oil, safflower oil, and flax oil. Avoid sugars and snack foods that contain salt and fat, such as potato chips, ice cream, candy, cookies, cake, breakfast cereals that are high in sugar, and sodas. Do not choose high-fat cheeses, sour cream, whole milk, butter, mayonnaise, fried foods, peanut butter (unless it is natural), or rich salad dressings. Do not drink alcoholic beverages at all—they are high in calories.

Here are some guidelines for balanced weight loss:

1. Eat three meals and two snacks daily to keep blood sugar levels stable.

2. Eat protein at each meal. Eat it in the form of lean meat, eggs, soy, and tofu. Include fish in your diet regularly.

3. Eat plenty of fruits and vegetables at each meal: five servings daily (½ cup is one serving).

4. Watch your portion sizes. A meal-sized serving of protein is about the size of your fist. Eat "two fists" of fruit, vegetables, and healthy grains at each meal. Eat "one thumb" of healthy fat at each meal.

5. Consume refined grains with caution. In some people, refined flour triggers binge eating.

6. Drink plenty of water daily.

To supplement a balanced, healthy weight-loss diet, you should increase the level of your routine exercise. You may also decide to investigate the inclusion of supplements such as green tea (which is theorized to burn up to 80 calories from fat, if taken with meals), chromium picolinate (to restore blood-sugar balance), L-tyrosine or kelp (for thyroid support and to raise serotonin levels), L-carnitine (to promote lean muscle), Relora (a patented product for stress-related weight gain), CLA (conjugated linoleic acid, which converts fats into muscle and energy), or chickweed (a natural appetite suppressant).

BASIC BRAIN FOOD

The key thing to remember about losing weight and maintaining weight loss is *balance*.

SUPPLEMENTAL BRAIN FOOD

An adjunct to a weight-loss eating plan could include supplements such as green tea, chromium picolinate, L-tyrosine or kelp, L-carnitine, Relora, CLA, or chickweed.

FOOD FOR THOUGHT

BRAIN-BUSTING TIP-OFF #37: Watch your portion sizes!

BRAIN-BOOSTING TIP #37: Eat three modest meals and two nutritious snacks every day to start losing weight and boost your brain at the same time.

chapter 38

BRAIN BALANCERS

I F YOU WANT to keep your mental edge and steer clear of roller-coaster moods, your brain needs continuing attention. Make sure you are feeding your brain all of the nutrients it needs to function at optimal levels every day and to safeguard yourself from the mental deterioration that can come from the aging process. Over time, your brain does not produce as many neurotransmitters as it once did. So you will want to do everything you can to supply it with all that it needs, especially when you experience stress. Eat modest portions of nutritious foods *regularly* to keep your brain supplied with fuel.

As I have repeated throughout this book, a key part of balanced nutrition for brain health is omega-3 fatty acids. Consuming omega-3 fatty acids can help reduce bad moods and improve scores on psychological tests.[1] In addition, omega-3 fatty acids and other essential fatty acids improve the health of your cardiovascular system, your nervous system, your skin health, your fat metabolism, and your joint flexibility. (They're not called "*essential* fatty acids" for nothing!)

Even if you eat plenty of oil-rich fish, the typical American diet does not supply the proper essential fatty acids on its own, so you must supplement your diet with them. Look for supplements that supply omega-3 oils derived from fish oil, flax oil, or borage oil. Please note that even though you will find most of these fatty acids in dark containers to keep out the light, they may go rancid quickly. This is especially true for flaxseed oil. If you cannot use a bottle of fish oil in a month, then purchase a smaller bottle and keep it in the refrigerator, or substitute fish oil capsules.

The B vitamins also play a key role in helping you to maintain peak brain health, along with ginkgo, which enhances neurotransmitter production, improves blood flow through your brain's capillaries, and helps your brain use glucose for energy production. Phosphatidyl serine (PS) helps to transmit nerve impulses from one cell to another and can help reduce various types of memory loss. Acetyl-L-carnitine

(ALC) helps to ease depression and helps cells fight free radicals and burn fat for energy. Huperzine A is derived from Chinese moss, and it helps your brain hang on to acetylcholine, which is a neurotransmitter vital to memory. A Chinese study found that huperzine A improved the mental functioning of Alzheimer's patients.

Exercise is another lesson in mind-body connection. A fit body contributes to a fit mind. Any type of exercise performed at least three times a week will help you stay fit. Exercise keeps your blood well supplied with oxygen by increasing your lung capacity and conditioning your heart. This will supercharge your brain. Exercise also causes your brain to produce more nerve growth factor, or NGF. Nerve growth factor helps brain cells to create branches that connect to fellow brain cells, so that information can be transferred speedily and accurately.

BASIC BRAIN FOOD

Eat lots of fish rich in omega-3 fatty acids, which is the best basic brain-balancing food of all.

SUPPLEMENTAL BRAIN FOOD

Key brain-balancing supplements include the B vitamins, ginkgo, phosphatidyl serine, acetyl-L-carnitine, and huperzine A.

FOOD FOR THOUGHT

BRAIN-BUSTING TIP-OFF #38: Your brain does not do well with a feast-or-famine lifestyle; eat at regular intervals.

BRAIN-BOOSTING TIP #38: Sprinkle flaxseeds on your oatmeal. They're rich in brain-boosting omega-3 fatty acids.

chapter 39

REPLENISH YOUR BRAIN

S OMETIMES, YOUR DEPLETED, overstressed brain just needs to be replenished, and you need to pull together the nutritional and supplemental information you have learned and apply it. In essence, you develop a personal plan for brain health, concentrating on bringing your brain back to a healthy state.

As I mentioned in chapter 5, I recommend that you supplement with GABA (gamma-aminobutyric acid), especially at the initial stage of brain replenishment, since the amino acid GABA affects your mind, memory, mood, and behavior, and because stress, trauma, and anxiety deplete your supply of GABA. GABA has a natural calming effect, and it helps to "cool" the brain. Remember that amino acid deficiencies occur when you experience long periods of pain, stress, depression, or anxiety. Once depletion occurs, your brain is then overwhelmed by anxiety signals, which leaves you tense and out of control. Your brain needs more than 100 mg of GABA to restore it to the proper level. I recommend capsules over tablets for easier assimilation.

Serotonin is a key neurotransmitter in brain function that enhances focus, elevates mood, and reduces anger and aggression. It can also help reduce cravings for carbohydrates and alcohol. You can also increase your serotonin level by simply eating certain carbohydrates such as whole-grain breads or cereals, pasta, potatoes, popcorn, or rice. These cause your body to produce insulin, which allows tryptophan to enter your brain; tryptophan is used by your body to create more of the neurotransmitter serotonin that will calm you down.[1]

Low magnesium levels are found in people with hyperirritability, depression, and anxiety. Magnesium is important to the proper metabolism of GABA. Because magnesium is such a vital mineral, enhancing the action and effect of amino acids, you need to find out if you need more of it. As I listed in chapter 5, the symptoms of magnesium deficiency include depression, fatigue, irregular heart-beat, irritable bowel syndrome and spastic symptoms, headaches, noise sensitivity, fibromyalgia, low blood sugar, dizziness, constipation, asthma, and chronic pain. If you supplement with magnesium, take 400 mg at bedtime. In addition to its other benefits, magnesium helps your muscles to relax. You can obtain extra magnesium by eating avocados, spinach, almonds, dark chocolate, and pumpkin or sunflower seeds.

To replenish your tired brain, take a good B-complex formula that contains vitamin B_6 and the full spectrum of B vitamins. Make sure you're getting plenty of vitamin C in the foods you eat and vitamin D through regular outdoor exercise; a little sunlight goes a long way.

Most important of all, eat a moderate, balanced, nutritionally sound diet every single day.

BASIC BRAIN FOOD

Obtain extra magnesium, vital to brain replenishment, by eating avocados, spinach, almonds, dark chocolate, and pumpkin or sunflower seeds.

SUPPLEMENTAL BRAIN FOOD

For brain replenishment, supplement with GABA, magnesium, and vitamins, especially the B-complex vitamins.

FOOD FOR THOUGHT

BRAIN-BUSTING TIP-OFF #39: Your brain health will *not* take care of itself; take steps to replenish your brain if it has been depleted by a stressful lifestyle.

BRAIN-BOOSTING TIP #39: To replenish your brain, increase your serotonin level by eating whole-grain breads or cereals, pasta, potatoes, popcorn, or rice.

SECTION 5

YOUR HEALTHY BRAIN

chapter 40

SHAKE OUT THE SUGAR!

DO YOU REACH for sugar in times of stress, depression, or anxiety? Sugar is especially detrimental to your brain and body function. Excessive sugar also suppresses your body's immune response. If you are consuming too much sugar on a daily basis, you may be setting yourself up for high blood sugar or diabetes. It would be wise for you to work to balance your blood sugar now, because low blood sugar can predispose you to develop diabetes later in your life. Diabetes occurs when the sugar and carbohydrates that a person consumes are not used properly by his or her body. Sooner or later, the person's pancreas no longer produces insulin, creating high blood sugar, which can be very dangerous.

In addition to diabetes, excessive sugar consumption leads to high cholesterol and triglycerides (therefore increased risk of atherosclerosis), excessive mood swings and food cravings (especially for women before menstruation), tooth decay, and gum disease. Even small blood sugar fluctuations disturb a person's sense of well-being. Large fluctuations caused by consuming too much sugar cause feelings of depression, anxiety, mood swings, fatigue, and even aggressive behavior.

Do you have a family history of diabetes? Do you crave sweets at certain times of the day or when you are under stress? Do you consume ice cream, chocolate, pies, cakes, and candy more than twice a week? Do you crave sodas or other sweetened drinks? Do you feel weak and shaky if your meal is delayed? Do you feel tense, uptight, and nervous at certain times during the day? Have you been choosing low-fat foods while ignoring the higher sugar content typically found in them?

If these feelings are familiar to you and your food choices are loaded with sugar, you must focus on eating more fiber and protein foods at each meal and cutting back on simple sugar. Watch out for the following types of foods: all sweet-tasting desserts and snacks, all nondiet sodas, fruit drinks with added sugar, dried fruits such as raisins, frozen or canned fruits packed in sugar syrup, sweetened milk products, and all foods (whether sweet tasting or not) processed with sugar (look for "sugars" on the nutritional label). Substitute stevia extract for sugar. Don't reach for artificial sweeteners because they have been implicated in very serious side effects. To satisfy your occasional sweet tooth without the health risks of artificial sweeteners, you can also substitute (if your health permits) the following: honey, rice syrup, sucarat (a natural sweetener made from sugar cane juice; use with caution if you have a blood sugar imbalance), or fructose (sugar derived from fruit).

Add fiber to your diet (brown rice, for example). It is very important for you to have a high-protein snack between meals, and you might want to try having a protein shake each morning. This will keep your blood sugar levels stable all day long.

True, limiting (and especially eliminating) sugar will not be easy to achieve. But for you to rebuild your brain and body, your sugar consumption *must* be curtailed. The following supplements can help you make the adjustment: chromium picolinate, B-complex vitamins, vitamin C, pantothenic acid, adrenal gland supplement, calcium, and magnesium.

By combining low-glycemic foods such as fiber foods together with exercise, amino acid supplementation, and nutritional supplements that help balance your blood sugar, you can optimize your brain's biochemistry.

BASIC BRAIN FOOD

Substitute the herbal supplement stevia for sugar.

SUPPLEMENTAL BRAIN FOOD

Supplements that can help you balance your blood sugar include chromium picolinate, B-complex vitamins, vitamin C, pantothenic acid, adrenal gland supplement, calcium, and magnesium.

FOOD FOR THOUGHT

BRAIN-BUSTING TIP-OFF #40: Excessive sugar is a brain-buster—lower your sugar consumption as soon as possible—today!

BRAIN-BOOSTING TIP #40: You can balance your blood sugar and boost your brain's biochemistry by sticking to a low-sugar, high-fiber, and high-protein diet.

chapter 41

SWEET DREAMS

Insomnia robs your brain of the essential downtime it needs to keep your body's systems running smoothly. A well-rested brain is a healthy brain, and sleep is a supreme tonic. Therefore, it is important that you get deep and restorative sleep every night.

If you have trouble getting to sleep at night or trouble staying asleep all night long, you have insomnia. If you have insomnia, it is vital to determine and change the cause of it. If you are thinking of taking prescription sleep aids, you should know that sleeping pills impair calcium absorption, are habit forming, and may paralyze the part of your brain that controls dreaming. As a result, many times sleeping pills can impair your clarity of thought and leave you feeling less than rested.

When you are working at reestablishing a healthy sleep pattern, take a hard look at your diet. Are you consuming caffeinated items such as coffee, tea, sodas, or chocolate? Caffeine is a stimulant, and it will keep you awake. What are you consuming in the evening? Sleep doesn't interfere with digestion—but digestion does interfere with sleep!

Here is a short list of suggested foods that will help you sleep: plain yogurt, a small bowl of oatmeal, a small serving of lean turkey, a banana, a small serving of tuna, a few whole-grain crackers. Everybody thinks of turkey as a source of tryptophan when they think of a natural sleep inducer, but did you know that tryptophan will work better when your stomach is *not* full, and it works better in combination with some complex carbohydrates? If you're about to go to bed, your body does not appreciate a protein overload. So if you are looking for the best midevening, sleep-promoting snack, take one slice of lean turkey and enjoy it on a slice of whole-grain bread.

I do not recommend sleep-inducing drugs because of their side effects, but there are natural sleep aids that may help you get to sleep and stay asleep. Passionflower is an antispasmodic sedative that helps to relax your mind and muscles. You can take it in tincture form (30 drops) or capsule form (500 mg) thirty minutes before you turn in for the night. Valerian helps anxiety-related sleep disorders. Valerian has a strong odor that many people object to, and some people may feel groggy or experience a "hangover effect" from it. If this happens to you, passionflower may be a better choice to help improve your sleep. Be careful not to combine valerian or passionflower with tranquilizers or antidepressant medications. Valerian also comes in tincture or capsule form. Take 30–60 drops or a 300–500 mg tablet thirty to sixty minutes before bedtime.

Several other natural supplements may also have beneficial effects: hops, melatonin, DHEA, L-theanine, calcium, magnesium, and inositol (enhances REM [rapid eye movement] sleep, the stage of deep sleep at which dreaming occurs).

Stop compromising the health of your body and brain and banish sleeplessness for good.

BASIC BRAIN FOOD

Sleep is the supreme tonic for your brain's health; specific foods can help or hinder your ability to sleep.

SUPPLEMENTAL BRAIN FOOD

To help you get good sleep, try one of these supplements (see chapter 36 for more ideas): hops, melatonin, DHEA, L-theanine.

FOOD FOR THOUGHT

BRAIN-BUSTING TIP-OFF #41: Avoid sleep-inducing drugs; try natural sleep inducers first.

BRAIN-BOOSTING TIP #41: "Brainy" bedtime snack suggestions include plain yogurt, oatmeal, a small serving of lean turkey, a banana, a small serving of tuna, or a few whole-grain crackers.

chapter 42

HORMONAL HARMONY:
PMS AND PREMENOPAUSE

FROM THE CRADLE to the grave, a woman's hormones play a vitally important role in her health and well-being—so much so that hundreds of books have been written on the topic. In this chapter and the next, I'm going to discuss the effects of hormones and a woman's brain and body. You may think you've heard it all before, but what you may not know is that the levels of hormones in your body are influenced by a number of important neurotransmitters in your brain. When neurotransmitters are out of balance, it becomes harder for your body to maintain proper hormone levels. Therefore, balancing your neurotransmitters often helps to balance your hormones by improving the communication between your brain and the glands that produce hormones in your body. The best way to balance neurotransmitters through your diet is by including adequate amounts of protein, carbohydrates, and fats while avoiding alcohol, caffeine, and nicotine. Now, let's discuss the times in women's lives when balancing hormones seems the most difficult—during premenopause and premenstrual stages.

It has been observed that 90 percent of premenopausal women suffer from some degree of premenstrual syndrome (PMS). The symptoms—which include mood swings, headaches, acne, bloating, irritability, fatigue, tender breasts, anxiety, depression, low back pain, and more—can last from two days to as long as two weeks, and are caused by the hormonal shift in estrogen and progesterone levels during the menstrual cycle.

In brief, PMS results from inadequate levels of progesterone in the second half of the menstrual cycle. This creates an "estrogen dominant" situation. Estrogen dominance occurs more often because of xenoestrogens such as environmental pollutants, pesticides, plastic-lined cans, stress, and foods (in particular, beef, poultry, and milk) laden with growth hormones. In addition, a diet that contains too

much salt, caffeine, sugar, and red meat are all implicated in the development of PMS. It has been found that many PMS sufferers also have
deficiencies in the B vitamins and in minerals.

The following recommendations will provide your body with nutrition and supplemental support necessary for relief of symptoms of PMS:

- Your diet should be low in fat and should include regular
  seafood consumption. Be sure to eat plenty of cruciferous
  vegetables (broccoli, cauliflower) and dark, leafy greens
  to reduce estrogen buildup. Prepare brown rice often to
  obtain B vitamins. Drink plenty of fresh, pure water.
- Buy organic meats, milk, milk products, and canned
  foods. Eliminate dairy products completely during your
  premenstrual days. Use whole grains, and keep your diet
  low in sugar and salt. Avoid caffeine and animal products
  as much as possible.
- Get more fiber in your diet naturally by choosing foods
  that are high in fiber such as beans and legumes (navy
  beans, kidney beans, black beans, pinto beans, lima beans,
  white beans, great northern beans, soybeans, split peas,
  lentils, chickpeas), fresh fruits and vegetables, with skins/
  peels where possible (prunes, artichokes, sweet potatoes,
  green peas, pears, apples, bananas, oranges, parsnips,
  potatoes), whole grains such as bulgar or barley, whole-
  grain pastas and whole-grain breads (wheat, millet, rye,
  etc.), nuts (especially almonds), and raw bran or oat bran
  cereals and baked products.
- Split your daily meals into many small meals taken
  throughout the day. To help control premenstrual cravings for sweets (mainly chocolate and refined sugar),
  increased appetite, headaches, and fatigue, consider the
  following supplements: balanced B-complex vitamin (50–
  100 mg of each B vitamin), chromium picolinate (at least
  200 mg daily), calcium (800–1,200 mg daily), magnesium
  (400–800 mg daily).
- To balance your estrogen/progesterone ratio, use a natural
  progesterone cream applied topically twice daily for two
  weeks prior to the expected beginning of your menstrual
  period.

- To ease your water retentiveness (which is why you have breast tenderness, bloating, and headaches), eliminate caffeine and chocolate. You can also use evening primrose oil (3,000 mg daily) and ginkgo biloba. To relieve lower back pain, take quercetin (1,000 mg) or bromelain (1,500 mg), or use ginger packs.

These recommendations may take two or three full monthly cycles to take full effect. You will need to be consistent in applying the changes to your diet in order to maintain your improvement.

BASIC BRAIN FOOD

To keep your energy up, split your daily meals into many small meals taken throughout the day.

SUPPLEMENTAL BRAIN FOOD

To help control premenstrual cravings for sweets, increased appetite, headaches, and fatigue, take a balanced B-complex vitamin, chromium picolinate, calcium, and magnesium.

FOOD FOR THOUGHT

BRAIN-BUSTING TIP-OFF #42: To lessen PMS symptoms, avoid sugar, caffeine, and milk products.

BRAIN-BOOSTING TIP #42: To keep your brain and body balanced during PMS, eat a high-fiber, high-protein, low-salt, and low-sugar diet.

chapter 43

HORMONAL HARMONY: MENOPAUSE

FROM ABOUT THE age of forty onward, most women are moving through what is known as perimenopause, followed by menopause, when menstrual periods cease altogether. During this stage of life, many women experience a decrease or even a cessation in their progesterone production because of irregular ovarian cycling and ovarian aging. At the same time, estrogen levels may be excessively or moderately high, causing a troubling, continual state of imbalance. The brain depends on healthy levels of both progesterone and estrogen in order to function at its best.

Women in perimenopause and menopause may experience a plethora of symptoms, some for years on end. These may include mood swings, fatigue, breast tenderness, foggy thinking, irritability, headaches, insomnia, decreased sex drive, anxiety, depression, allergy symptoms, fat gain, hair loss, memory loss, water retention, bone loss, slow metabolism, endometrial and breast cancers, and many more. In other words, hormonal imbalance has far-reaching effects on many tissues in the body, including the brain, heart and blood vessels, bones, uterus, and breasts.

Menopause can vary widely between individuals. Many factors influence the timing of menopause, including trauma, surgery, and body weight. Physically active and well-nourished women experience late menopause, while smokers experience earlier menopause.

The key to a smooth transition is bringing the levels of estrogen and progesterone back into balance as well as managing stress. To bring the hormone levels back into balance, I recommend using natural progesterone cream. Natural progesterone has been found to be effective in combating perimenopausal anxiety and mood swings. In addition, it plays a very important part in the prevention and reversal of osteoporosis. Natural progesterone offers a woman all of these benefits without hormone replacement therapy (HRT).

Natural progesterone is part of a menopausal protocol that helps women live rich lives without hormone replacement therapy, part of a natural transition that also includes dietary changes and supplements.

When a woman is young, her body makes ample hormones to keep her young, healthy, and vibrant. As the years pass, her body does not produce hormones in balanced amounts, but she can turn to the plant kingdom, where natural hormones abound. Soybeans, black cohosh, Mexican wild yam, and licorice can be of benefit to a perimenopausal/menopausal woman.

But for many women, stressful lifestyles have made it necessary to move up to bioidentical hormones that are derived from these plants and then synthesized in a lab to be molecularly similar to the hormones our bodies make—estrogen, progesterone, DHEA, and so forth. (This is unlike synthetic hormones, which the drug companies purposely make different in order to patent drugs such as Prempro, Provera, and Premarin.)

Bioidentical hormones are much safer for your body because they are easier for your body to metabolize without many of the side effects that synthetic hormones create. They have been shown to increase your energy, improve your sense of well-being, improve your memory, aid weight loss, increase libido, and reduce facial hair. Conversely, synthetic hormones have side effects that include lack of sex drive, poor sleep, increased cancer risk, and weight gain.

Now, neither bioidentical hormones nor synthetic hormones can do the whole job alone. You must clean up your diet, eat sensibly and often, get plenty of rest, drink plenty of water, and take a calcium supplement and a good daily multivitamin, taking particular concern for the health of your adrenal glands, because they play an important role in your hormone balance.

You should follow these dietary guidelines to help ease the symptoms of menopause: add soy foods to your diet; limit sugar, sodium, caffeine, pies, cakes, and pastries; limit red meat; eat fresh vegetables, fruits, and nuts; instead of three large meals a day, eat several smaller meals throughout the day; limit dairy products; try adding seaweed to your diet—Nori, Wakame, Kombu, and Arame contain natural hormones and plant chemicals to help you during menopause;[1] and eat more melons, bananas, dried fruits such as apricots and figs, and citrus fruits like oranges and lemons, which are high in potassium. Potassium-rich foods help balance sodium and water retention.[2]

In addition to dietary changes, be sure to make some important lifestyle changes that bring you a daily dose of exercise, laughter, and relaxation.

There are also many natural herbal remedies that can alleviate your menopause symptoms and help you find balance in this season of life. I suggest that you try them one by one and determine for yourself the ones that really give you comfort: black cohosh, black currant seed oil, dong quai (high in phytoestrogens), bioflavonoids (also high in phytoestrogens), licorice (for your adrenal health), plant enzymes (taken with meals), red raspberry, vitamin B-complex, vitamin C, vitamin E (normalizes hormones), 5-HTP (for insomnia and anxiety at night).

If you do your best to maintain your physical, mental, and emotional balance through the middle season of your life, the process of aging will be more graceful and less painful for you.

BASIC BRAIN FOOD

You'll never go wrong if you eat plenty of fresh vegetables, fruits, nuts, and fish.

SUPPLEMENTAL BRAIN FOOD

Circumstances may require a woman to take bioidentical hormones, which are derived from plants and synthesized in a lab to be molecularly similar to natural hormones.

FOOD FOR THOUGHT

BRAIN-BUSTING TIP-OFF #43: Women in midlife should limit sugar, sodium, dietary fats, caffeine, red meat, and dairy products.

BRAIN-BOOSTING TIP #43: Soybeans, Mexican wild yam, licorice, and black cohosh can help balance a woman's hormones, which leads to better brain health.

chapter 44

HORMONAL HARMONY: ANDROPAUSE ("MALE MENOPAUSE")

WHILE EVERYONE KNOWS that women journey through meno-pause and all of its life-disrupting symptoms, men's bodies are experiencing hormonal changes as well. As testosterone production decreases, men's cognitive function declines, they feel less vital and less virile, they experience loss of muscle mass and strength, their energy declines, and their hairline recedes or disappears completely. For men, this lesser-known physiological change is known as *andropause*, or male menopause.

This is a very real physiological condition, and it is very unsettling to most men. It has been estimated by some researchers that currently as many as 2.5 million American men between the ages of forty and fifty-five are experiencing signs and symptoms of andropause. Most of these physical, mental, and emotional changes take place over the course of ten to fifteen years.

A man may notice that his eight hours of uninterrupted sleep become a thing of the past as he makes his way to the bathroom in the middle of the night due to increased urinary frequency. Abdominal fat now replaces a formerly well-toned stomach, and his libido starts to fade along with his hairline.

The importance of testosterone cannot be stressed enough. It plays a vital role in a male's sense of well-being. It has a positive effect on cholesterol levels, bone density, muscle mass, protein breakdown, and maintenance of secondary sex characteristics such as libido, facial and body hair, and more. With low testosterone, your symptoms may include an inability to concentrate and memory failure (lower cognitive function in general); irritability; general tiredness, weakness, and passivity; diminished sex drive; and depression, moodiness, and anxiety.

These symptoms can be turned around with testosterone supplementation. A recent study revealed the effects of testosterone supplementation on ten men, aged sixty to seventy-five, in a double-blind trial. The results were impressive. Testosterone supplements improved exercise endurance time, increased fat-free mass (i.e., muscle), and improved balance.[1] A very important fact for men to note is that rebalancing testosterone and estrogen (yes, men have estrogen too) seems to provide protection against hormone-related cancers to which both men and women are more prone when their bodies have an excess of estrogen in comparison with other hormones.

Can your diet help? Yes, it can. For starters, take a look at your weight. If you are overweight, your body will produce too much estrogen. Lose weight. Fat cells, especially in the abdominal area, produce aromatase enzyme, which converts testosterone to estrogen. Also make sure you are getting enough zinc (80–90 mg daily), since zinc functions as a natural aromatase inhibitor. Food sources of zinc include oysters, red meat, poultry, beans, nuts, and dairy. You should reduce or eliminate alcohol from your diet to enable your liver to better remove excess estrogen.

To boost your testosterone naturally, you can try a combination of chrysin (a flavonoid, or plant pigment; take one 1,500 mg. capsule daily), muira puama (a plant extract; take one 850 mg capsule daily), and urtica dioica (a plant root extract; take one 200 mg capsule daily). The chrysin will block the aromatase enzyme from converting testosterone to estrogen, and the plant extracts will reduce the conversion process, thereby boosting overall levels of free testosterone naturally.[2]

BASIC BRAIN FOOD

If you are a male in midlife, you may be able to alleviate some symptoms of male menopause through hormonal and nutritional supplementation.

SUPPLEMENTAL BRAIN FOOD

Men: consider testosterone replacement therapy as well as the three natural testosterone-boosters: chrysin, muira puama, and urtica dioica.

FOOD FOR THOUGHT

Brain-Busting Tip-Off #44: Eliminate alcohol from your diet to better enable your liver to eliminate excess estrogen.

Brain-Boosting Tip #44: To balance your brain and your testosterone, increase your intake of zinc-rich foods such as oysters, red meat, and other high-protein foods.

chapter 45

B IS FOR BRAIN BOOSTING

ERTAIN NUTRIENTS AND chemical compounds are more essential to your brain's health than others, and the B vitamins are high on that list. So are all antioxidants, which you obtain from including fresh, bright-colored fruits and vegetables on your daily menu.

It has become clear that careful attention to your nutrition can help prevent the cognitive decline that we usually attribute to growing older. Your neurons need a good supply of nutrients in order to keep communications pathways flowing. Here is a summary of what I mean:

> Neurons that can't get their messages through signaling pathways are like cell phones that can't get their signals through to other cell phones. Why does this happen?
>
> As the brain matures, cell division becomes largely restricted to specific regions of the brain, and brain cells tend to become more vulnerable to two partners in crime: oxidative stress and inflammation.... The brain is thought to be especially vulnerable to oxidative stress.
>
> Weighing just 3 pounds, the brain accounts for only 2 percent of the body's total mass, yet it uses up to half of the body's total oxygen consumed during mental activity, [according to James Joseph, neuroscientist with the USDA-Agricultural Research Service Human Nutrition Research Center on Aging at Tufts University of Boston]. Phytochemicals [chemical compounds derived from plants], together with essential nutrients in foods, provide a health-benefits cocktail of sorts.[1]

Researcher Joseph goes on to say, "A partial measure of the antioxidant effect is called 'ORAC,' for Oxygen Radical Absorbance Capacity. ORAC scores are now showing up in charts and on some food and beverage packages. They may be helpful in choosing foods to include in your diet."[2] Foods that rank high on the ORAC measure include cooked artichokes, pecans, walnuts, and raw asparagus. Almost all other fruits and vegetables also provide antioxidant protection for your brain and body.

Many of those same foods also provide the "Big B" for your brain—the B vitamins. The family of B vitamins includes thiamine (B_1), riboflavin (B_2), niacin (B_3), pantothenic acid and biotin (B_5), and vitamins B_6 and B_{12}.

B_1, commonly known as thiamine, is known as the "morale vitamin" because of its beneficial effect on your mental stability and memory. It is also crucial to the health of your nervous system. If your diet is high in carbohydrates, then B_1 is absolutely essential. B_1 improves food assimilation, thereby stabilizing your appetite.

B_2, which is known as riboflavin, is a water-soluble vitamin that is easily absorbed through the small intestines. It plays an important part in many chemical reactions in your body.

Niacin, or B_3, assists in the functioning of your digestive system, and it helps to maintain the health of your skin and nerves. It is important for the conversion of food to energy.

Pantothenic acid, also called biotin or B_5, is a blessing when a person is under stress. It has an enhancing and beneficial effect upon the adrenal glands, whose proper functioning is crucial when a person is under stressful conditions.

B_6 may have the greatest effect on the immune system of all the B vitamins, because a deficiency can result in a vast array of immune-response problems and has been linked to tumor growth. A lack of B_6 makes the size of the thymus—the gland that produces T-cells—decrease in size. B_6 should not be taken by itself; it must be taken with amino acids.

B_{12} is also known as cobalamin, and on the molecular level, it is the most complex of all the B group. It is required by your body for the formation of red blood cells, which are needed to prevent mood-sapping fatigue and low energy. Vitamin B_{12} is crucial too for your body because it helps your system process fats.

Neither humans nor animals can manufacture B_{12} in their bodies, which must be combined with calcium for proper absorption. Many people have a hard time absorbing B_{12} from the foods they eat, and vegetarian foods are lacking in this important vitamin, so I recommend that everyone take a daily dose of B-complex in order to obtain the B_{12} they need. Take a B-complex formula that contains the full spectrum of B vitamins.

To get B vitamins from your food, include more of the following foods in your diet:

- *Thiamine (vitamin B_1)* is found in fortified breads, cereals, pasta, whole grains (especially wheat germ), lean meats (especially pork), fish, dried beans, peas, and soybeans.
- *Riboflavin (vitamin B_2)* is found in lean meats, eggs, legumes, nuts, green leafy vegetables, and dairy products. Breads and cereals are often fortified with riboflavin.
- *Niacin (vitamin B_3)* is found in dairy products, poultry, fish, lean meats, nuts, and eggs. Legumes and enriched breads and cereals also supply some niacin.
- *Vitamin B_5 (pantothenic acid, biotin)* is found in eggs, fish, milk and milk products, whole-grain cereals, legumes, yeast, broccoli and other vegetables in the cabbage family, white and sweet potatoes, and lean beef.
- *Vitamin B_6* is found in beans, nuts, legumes, eggs, meats, fish, whole grains, and fortified breads and cereals.
- *Vitamin B_{12}* is found in eggs, meat, poultry, shellfish, milk, and milk products.[3]

BASIC BRAIN FOOD

The family of B vitamins is the big B for brain health.

SUPPLEMENTAL BRAIN FOOD

Take a good B-complex supplement daily.

FOOD FOR THOUGHT

BRAIN-BUSTING TIP-OFF #45: As you age, pay more attention, not less, to obtaining B vitamins and antioxidants through the foods you choose.

BRAIN-BOOSTING TIP #45: Boost your brain with lots of antioxidants found in brightly colored fruits and vegetables.

chapter 46

FOOD FOR YOUR AGING BRAIN

As I MENTIONED in the previous chapter, your brain needs a steady supply of antioxidants, B vitamins, and other nutrients as you grow older. If you pay attention to your nutritional intake and augment your diet wisely with hormone replacement and age-specific supplements, your aging brain can and will rebuild and restore itself and remain sharp and healthy for years to come. To add years to your life, follow these basic dietary guidelines:

- Avoid fried foods, red meat, too much caffeine, and highly spiced and processed foods.
- Eat fresh seafood at least twice weekly.
- Have a "green drink" daily (wheat grass, barley green).
- Include nuts, seeds, beans, fiber, and essential fatty acids in your diet.
- Eat lots of fresh fruits and vegetables (full of enzymes, vitamins, minerals, and fiber).

Don't fall prey to your slower metabolism and a sedentary lifestyle. Keep moving and begin now to practice caloric reduction. As you age, your body requires fewer calories; it burns calories at a lower rate. A low-calorie diet has been shown to protect your DNA from damage. Having healthy DNA will help prevent organ and tissue degeneration. Try to get more "bang for your caloric buck" by eating only high-quality, densely nutritious foods at each meal. For example choose to eat *fresh* fruit and vegetables, organically grown if possible.

If you were to eliminate the water and fat from your body, 75 percent of what would remain would be protein. Muscles, cell membranes, enzymes, and the neurotransmitters are all proteins. Proteins are made up of amino acids. Therefore, amino acids become another vital contributor to the health of all of your cell functions, especially those of your brain.

Besides making sure that you include good sources of lean protein in your daily diet, you may also decide to replenish your brain with amino acid supplements. Here are some to consider:

- *L-theanine* (an amino acid found in green tea, helps calm and restore; increases GABA)
- *Lysine* (effective in the natural treatment of hypothyroidism, Alzheimer's disease, and Parkinson's disease)
- *Glutamine* (a prime brain nutrient and energy source. Supplementing your brain with glutamine may rapidly improve memory, recall, concentration, and alertness.)
- *Tyrosine* (an antioxidant and a source of quick energy, especially for the brain. Tyrosine also helps to build your body's natural supply of adrenaline and thyroid hormones.)
- *Glycine* (converts to creatine in your body to retard nerve and muscle degeneration and helps to control hypoglycemic sugar drops)
- *Taurine* (a neurotransmitter that stabilizes your nervous system, a potent antiseizure amino acid)

For the best uptake and absorption, you should take amino acids with their nutrient cofactors such as vitamin B_6 and vitamin C. It's best to take amino acid supplements in the morning, before meals, or between meals so they won't compete for absorption with amino acids in foods. Make sure to take them with plenty of water for optimum absorption.

BASIC BRAIN FOOD

Nuts, seeds, beans, and fresh produce feed a healthy brain.

SUPPLEMENTAL BRAIN FOOD

For brain health, consider taking amino acid supplements: L-theanine, lysine, glutamine, tyrosine, glycine, and taurine.

FOOD FOR THOUGHT

BRAIN-BUSTING TIP-OFF #46: For better absorption of amino acids from the foods you eat, don't take amino acid supplements with your meals.

BRAIN-BOOSTING TIP #46: Eat fresh seafood at least twice weekly to help minimize the effects of aging on your brain.

chapter 47

ENERGY TO SPARE

EVERYONE LOVES TO feel energetic and full of life. Sometimes, though, we sabotage ourselves when it comes to improving and sustaining our energy level all day long, especially because of the food choices we make.

What is the single best nutritional decision you can make today to ensure that you will open your front door tomorrow and walk into your day with a brisk, bouncy step? That's easy—*eat breakfast.* Study after study has shown that people who eat breakfast have more energy all day long. Breakfast skippers may declare they "just don't feel like eating" first thing in the morning, but they probably overeat as the day goes on in an effort to compensate for the lack of fuel their bodies need. Skipping breakfast makes it difficult to achieve mental focus.

"Not eating breakfast basically puts your entire day in jeopardy—it's like running your car without oil and gas—using the drudge at the bottom of the gas tank," says nutrition expert Elizabeth Somer.[1]

You don't have to prepare a breakfast of bacon and eggs and pancakes. In fact, it would be a lot better if you didn't. Just eat a container of low-fat yogurt and a piece of whole-grain toast or a banana and a handful of almonds. Then proceed through the rest of your day choosing foods that will enhance your energy, not sap it.

You should be sure to consume quality protein at every meal. This will help to give you the energy you need, and it will provide your body with slow- and even-burning fuel throughout the day. Sources of good-quality protein include low-fat dairy and soy products, fish, lean chicken and turkey, beans, nuts, and seeds. One 6-ounce portion of lean chicken provides your body with a whopping 85 grams of protein. Fish is also a concentrated source of protein, providing about 41.2 grams per serving. An 8-ounce container of yogurt (depending on the type) will give you 8 to 13 grams of protein, and a half a cup of tofu, about 10.1 grams.[2] Ideally, adults need 7 to 9 grams of protein for every 20 pounds of their body weight.[3] So if you weigh 150 pounds, you need to eat about 50 grams of protein daily to stay healthy. (If you don't get enough protein, your body starts to break down its own tissues.)

Protein sources contain tyrosine, the amino acid that helps produce neurotransmitters that keep you mentally alert. Tyrosine helps to build the body's natural supply of adrenaline and thyroid hormones. It is also an antioxidant and is a source of quick energy, especially for the brain.

To keep yourself energized, also be sure to stay adequately hydrated. Sometimes you don't really need any food; the only boost you actually need is a glass or a bottle of water. If you drink plenty of water, both your energy and your mood will improve.

Your water requirements may vary depending on your activity level and your environment. Your home and work environment, which is likely to be heated in winter and air-conditioned in summer, may dehydrate you more quickly than you realize, especially if you live at a high altitude or in a dry climate or both.

A final suggestion: for more even energy and mood throughout your demanding day, you might want to try eating a number of smaller meals, or modest meals interspersed with nourishing snacks, instead of the typical American "three square meals a day," or skipping meals.

BASIC BRAIN FOOD

The average person needs about 50 grams of protein per day.

SUPPLEMENTAL BRAIN FOOD

No supplement can substitute for good protein and pure water.

FOOD FOR THOUGHT

BRAIN-BUSTING TIP-OFF #47: Don't wait until you get thirsty—stay well-hydrated all day long.

BRAIN-BOOSTING TIP #47: Eat a good breakfast every single day for optimum brain function.

chapter 48

OUTLOOK IS EVERYTHING

Y OUR BODY MAY be in optimum condition, but if your outlook is glum and grim, your mental health needs a boost, and your brain is telling you that it needs some mood-boosting food. You can help to make sure that your low times are temporary by making good nutritional choices.

Carbohydrates—if they are complex carbohydrates—boost your brain's serotonin levels, and serotonin is known as the "good mood" chemical. Choose whole-grain breads, brown rice, beans, and fresh vegetables instead of processed, refined carbohydrates such as white breads and white rice. Avoid carbohydrates such as candy, sweet baked goods, and junk foods, even if they are the only things available in the vending machine at work. Those are simple carbohydrates, and their sugar content alone will give you a temporary "buzz," only to let you down badly later.

Instead of playing with your blood sugar levels, keep them even by eating smart. Leave that cookie for someone else. Instead, try some air-popped popcorn, fresh fruit, or whole-grain crackers.

Many people who suffer from low moods are deficient in folic acid. You can eat specific foods that will supply you with extra folic acid. Choose foods such as asparagus; avocados; garbanzos, soybeans, and other beans; lentils and other legumes; oranges; broccoli; and spinach and its dark leafy cousins. Magnesium relaxes your tense muscles. Here again, avocados and spinach can help. You can also get magnesium from dark chocolate (preferably in small servings), almonds, and pumpkin or sunflower seeds.

I mentioned niacin (also known as B_3) in chapter 45, where I described the valuable B vitamins in detail. Niacin assists in the functioning of your digestive system, and it keeps your skin and nerves healthy. It is also important for the conversion of food to energy. Some experts believe that it can help alleviate depression, anxiety, or panic. Niacin is found in dairy products, poultry, fish, lean meats, brown rice, nuts, and eggs. Legumes and breads and cereals made with enriched grains also supply some niacin. Of course, these foods also supply you with some proteins, which also give you mood-boosting energy.

If you lack zinc in your diet, you will have a very short "fuse." You will be irritable and easily angered. For your own sake and for the sake of your family and the other people around you, see if you can improve your bad mood with some zinc-containing whole-grain bread, a glass of milk, an egg or two, or even some oysters.

The average American adult consumes more than twice as much sodium in a day than is recommended. This has the negative effect of making a person retain water, which makes him or her feel sluggish. It also causes blood pressure to rise, which is hard on every part of a person's body.

Most people should be limiting their sodium intake to about 1,300–2,000 mg per day (less for older people or those with specific health concerns). According to the *Harvard Health Letter*, the average adult consumes 3,000 to 4,000 mg of sodium per day.

Even mood-enhancing foods should not be eaten in large quantities, or you will have too much of a good thing. Don't let your low mood drive you to overeat. If you do, you will undo many of the effects of the good nutrition by raising your blood sugar and consequently your insulin and cortisone levels. You want your food to *enhance* your mood, not make it swing wildly back and forth.

Eat smart and eat healthy. Eat a well-balanced, nutritious diet that is made up mostly of an array of fresh vegetables and fruits, whole grains and nuts, healthy oils, minimal sugars, and well-chosen, lean protein, and you will help both your mood and your waistline. The foods and extra supplements that you consume cannot possibly cure everything that ails you, but they definitely can improve your mood.

BASIC BRAIN FOOD

Complex carbohydrates boost your brain's serotonin levels, and serotonin is the "good mood" chemical.

SUPPLEMENTAL BRAIN FOOD

Irritable? Try a zinc supplement, or eat zinc-containing foods such as whole-grain bread, milk, eggs, or oysters.

FOOD FOR THOUGHT

BRAIN-BUSTING TIP-OFF #48: Even though certain foods can improve your outlook, don't eat too *much* of the "good-for-you" foods—you might become overweight.

BRAIN-BOOSTING TIP #48: Dairy products, poultry, fish, lean meats, brown rice, nuts, eggs, legumes, and breads and cereals made with enriched grains supply both niacin and protein, which will give you a better outlook and more energy.

chapter 49

HOW TO MAKE EVERY DAY
A GOOD BRAIN DAY

MOST PEOPLE WOULD say that they'd rather have a good brain day than a good hair day! Each of us wants to stride through our days feeling our best mentally and physically. It makes such a huge difference in life. By applying the advice in this book, you can make every day a good brain day.

Feeling your very best means consuming personally balanced nutrition every single day. Each person is a little different, although there are certain common denominators, so you need to explore both the principles and the possibilities as you come up with a manageable, affordable, and sustainable nutrition plan that works for *you*.

It is so important to make a conscious effort to eat properly, because your body needs high-quality fuel in order to repair, rebuild, and regenerate itself. So many of the foods we Americans prefer actually sabotage our physical and mental and emotional health, instead of supplying high-quality nutrition for our bodies and minds.

One of the simplest things you can do is eat breakfast every day. Your brain needs glucose, and studies show that children and adults who skip breakfast do not perform as well on tests at school or tasks on the job.

Here is my personal eating plan. It is high in nutrition, yet it eliminates all the foods that can undermine my physical and mental health.

- *Upon rising*: One 8-ounce glass of water with juice from ½ fresh lemon, with stevia extract* to sweeten

- *Breakfast*: One of the following:
- One or two poached or hard-boiled eggs on a slice of millet bread
- Oatmeal or oat bran with 1 tablespoon Braggs Aminos*

- Buckwheat pancakes with a little butter or almond butter
- Millet toast with almond butter

- *Midmorning*: A glass of a green drink (liquid chlorophyll or Kyo-Green*), a cup of dandelion tea, or a bottle of water

- *Lunch*: One of the following:
- A fresh green salad with lemon and olive oil dressing
- An open-faced millet sandwich with mayonnaise, veggies, seafood, turkey, or chicken
- Vegetable soup with a slice of millet bread
- A chicken, tuna, or vegetable pasta salad

- *Midafternoon*: One of the following snacks:
- Rice crackers or baked corn chips with some rice cheese or soy cheese
- A bottle of water with a hard-boiled or deviled egg
- Raw veggies
  and
- A cup of green tea, sweetened with stevia*

- *Dinner*: One of the following:
- Baked, broiled, or poached fish or chicken or turkey with steamed brown rice
- Baked potato with Bragg Aminos*
- Rice with soy cheese
- An oriental stir-fry with brown rice and Braggs Aminos*
- A small omelet with a veggie filling (soy or rice cheese can be added)
- A vegetarian casserole
- A hot or cold vegetable pasta salad

- *Before bed*: A cup of herb tea such as dandelion or chamomile, sweetened with stevia*

*These supplements I've mentioned above are available at your local health food store: Kyo-Green (a complete green superfood that contains protein and all the B vitamins), stevia extract (also known as "sweet herb" [*Stevia rebaudiana*], stevia is twenty-five times sweeter than sugar and yet it balances the blood sugar and has antifungal properties; has zero calories; and, unlike sugar, does not promote tooth decay), and Braggs Amino Acids (a natural health alternative to soy sauce made from soybeans and purified water only—no additives or preservatives, no alcohol, no chemicals—that can be dashed or sprayed on salads, vegetables, rice and beans, tofu, casseroles and soups, potatoes, beans, fish, poultry, jerky, tempeh, gravies, sauces, and popcorn).

BASIC BRAIN FOOD

Using the information in this book, assemble your own personal nutrition plan to make every day a good brain day.

SUPPLEMENTAL BRAIN FOOD

Consider supplementing your daily diet with a green drink (liquid chlorophyll) daily.

FOOD FOR THOUGHT

BRAIN-BUSTING TIP-OFF #49: Don't let yourself lapse into the typical American diet or pace of life.

BRAIN-BOOSTING TIP #49: Know your own brain and body, and learn how to meet your personal nutritional needs as well as your needs for exercise and rest.

chapter 50

THE BRAIN-BOOSTING SHOPPING LIST

BY NOW YOU are well aware that as the control center of your body, your brain and its nourishment should be your top priority. Making healthy food choices that supply your brain with the right nutrients can improve your concentration, boost your memory, speed up your reaction times, sharpen your motor skills, help you de-stress, and slow down the aging process.

I hope this book has been helpful to you and provided you with information about the brain-body connection that will improve the quality of life for you and those you love. Use the following shopping list, compiled from all of the foods suggested in this book, in order to stock your kitchen with as many brain-boosting foods as you can. Obviously, you won't be purchasing everything on this list every time you go to the grocery store. Instead, use this list more like a master list of "approved" brain-boosting foods that will increase the health of your brain and body. The starred items (*) are what I call the "brain-boosting all-star team" because they directly affect and improve your brain's performance. The rest of the foods on this list relieve specific health conditions and therefore contribute to better brain function.

PRODUCE	
Apples	Mangos
Apricots	Melons
Artichokes	Mushrooms
Asparagus	Onions
Avocados*	Oranges
Bananas	Papayas
Blackberries	Parsnips

PRODUCE

Blueberries*	Pears
Broccoli	Peas
Brussels sprouts	Persimmons
Cabbage	Pineapples
Cantaloupe	Potatoes
Carrots	Prunes
Celery	Pumpkin
Cherries	Seaweed
Corn	Spinach*
Dates	Squash
Figs	Sweet peppers
Grapes	Sweet potatoes
Kale	Tomatoes
Kiwi	Turnips
Lemons	Watermelon
Lettuce	

DAIRY AND EGGS

Low-fat milk*	Soy cheese
Omega-3 eggs*	Yogurt, plain
Rice cheese	

MEATS, POULTRY, AND FISH

Free-range chicken	Shellfish
Duck	Shrimp
Flounder*	Tofu (preferred over red meat and pork)
Mackerel*	Tuna*
Oysters	Turkey
Salmon*	

NUTS AND SEEDS

Almonds*	Pumpkin seeds
Flaxseeds	Sesame seeds

NUTS AND SEEDS

Hazelnuts	Sunflower seeds
Pecans	Walnuts
Poppy seeds	

LEGUMES*

Baked beans	Lentils
Black beans	Lima beans
Black-eyed peas	Navy beans
Chickpeas (garbanzo beans)	Pinto beans
Great northern beans	Soybeans
Green beans	Split peas
Kidney beans	White beans

CONDIMENTS, SWEETENERS, AND SNACKS

Almond butter	Honey
Baked corn chips	Hot peppers
Blackstrap molasses	Maple syrup
Brown rice syrup	Olives (canned)
Butter	Popcorn
Dark chocolate*	Rice crackers
Garlic*	Stevia

FATS AND OILS

Flaxseed oil	Walnut oil
Olive oil	

WHOLE GRAINS*

Bran	Millet
Brown rice	Oats, oatmeal, oat bran
Barley	Quinoa
Buckwheat (kasha)	Rye
Bulgar	Sugar-free, whole-grain cereals fortified with iron and B vitamins

WHOLE GRAINS*	
Flax meal	Wheat bran
Hominy grits	Whole-grain pastas (all types)

BEVERAGES	
Dandelion tea	Mineral water
Distilled water	Rice milk
Green tea*	Soy milk
Herbal tea	

MISCELLANEOUS	
Bragg's Aminos	Green superfoods (Kyo-Green)
Brewer's yeast	Multivitamins
Green drinks (wheatgrass, barley green)	Protein shakes

BASIC BRAIN FOOD

Planning a shopping list ahead of time will help you avoid the temptation to purchase junk foods that can leave your brain and body depleted of important nutrients.

SUPPLEMENTAL BRAIN FOOD

Be sure to add multivitamins and a vitamin B-complex to your shopping list.

FOOD FOR THOUGHT

BRAIN-BUSTING TIP-OFF #50: Don't shop when you're hungry. You'll be more inclined to purchase unhealthy food choices.

BRAIN-BOOSTING TIP #50: Substitute as many brain-boosting foods into your diet as you can for improved brain function and overall health.

FIFTY BRAIN BOOSTERS AT A GLANCE

BRAIN-BOOSTING TIP #1: A smart start to a better brain is eating choline-rich eggs.

BRAIN-BOOSTING TIP #2: Pregnant women are nourishing two brains and should eat 60 grams of protein daily.

BRAIN-BOOSTING TIP #3: The nutrients, antibodies, enzymes, and hormones in breast milk make it the best brain food for your baby.

BRAIN-BOOSTING TIP #4: For simple brain nutrition, think "complex"— complex carbohydrates such as whole grains and legumes.

BRAIN-BOOSTING TIP #5: To help diffuse stress and its effects on your brain, go for fish, beans, kasha, millet, blackberries, broccoli, bananas, dates, watermelon, and almonds.

BRAIN-BOOSTING TIP #6: To keep your brain's neurotransmitters running at peak performance, eat a variety of fish often.

BRAIN-BOOSTING TIP #7: Brightly colored fruits and vegetables provide antioxidants that help protect your brain.

BRAIN-BOOSTING TIP #8: Dehydration impairs cognitive function, so be sure to drink eight to ten glasses of water per day.

BRAIN-BOOSTING TIP #9: Brain-friendly foods include lean meat, whole grains, beans, nuts, fresh fruits, and veggies.

BRAIN-BOOSTING TIP #10: Essential brain nutrients include the full range of vitamins and minerals.

BRAIN-BOOSTING TIP #11: Before your brain's limbic system detects your next hunger pang or craving, stock up on low-glycemic snack foods like grapes, strawberries, apples, and carrots to keep your blood sugar on an even keel.

BRAIN-BOOSTING TIP #12: When you feel stressed, take a popcorn break.

Brain-Boosting Tip #13: To manage stress and anxiety that drain your brain, eliminate common food stressors such as yeast, sugar, and dairy.

Brain-Boosting Tip #14: You can improve your mood more by eating a piece of whole-grain toast than by eating a candy bar.

Brain-Boosting Tip #15: Combine whole grains and proteins at meals to rid yourself of "brain drain" after a time of grief, conflict, prolonged pain, or depression.

Brain-Boosting Tip #16: If you are feeling depressed, boost your mood and your brain function by enjoying a high-protein shake.

Brain-Boosting Tip #17: Watch for unhealthy changes in teenage eating habits, and reinforce the importance of proper nutrition for a healthy brain and body now and in the future.

Brain-Boosting Tip #18: Counteract "brain clouds" and fatigue by eating mangoes, papayas, bananas, avocados, and pineapples to get extra plant enzymes from your food.

Brain-Boosting Tip #19: Eating folate-rich leafy vegetables such as spinach can safeguard against depression, as well as improve cognitive functioning.

Brain-Boosting Tip #20: For clearer thinking, avoid high-fat foods that will raise cholesterol, clog arteries, and limit the flow of blood to the brain.

Brain-Boosting Tip #21: Drinking more water may help alleviate the migraines some people experience when the brain begins to dehydrate.

Brain-Boosting Tip #22: Eating three additional servings of fruits and vegetables every day may reduce your risk of having a stroke.

Brain-Boosting Tip #23: To lower inflammation throughout your body and brain, eat more blueberries and kiwi fruit.

Brain-Boosting Tip #24: If you're feeling faint, eat fresh fruit or vegetables.

Brain-Boosting Tip #25: Iodine is needed for healthy brain and thyroid function; obtain it easily by using iodized salt, drinking milk, and eating shellfish and seaweed.

BRAIN-BOOSTING TIP #26: To fight chronic fatigue and improve brain functioning, stay as active as possible, starting with a short walk each day, but not so much that you get fatigued.

BRAIN-BOOSTING TIP #27: Eating a low-fat diet with plenty of fruits, vegetables, and whole grains can help you manage fibromyalgia.

BRAIN-BOOSTING TIP #28: Dietary changes can balance brain chemistry and reduce pain; start by eliminating starchy foods, sugars, artificial sweeteners, food colorings, and preservatives.

BRAIN-BOOSTING TIP #29: Enhance your brain health by eating sources of lecithin such as grains, legumes, fish, wheat germ, and brewer's yeast.

BRAIN-BOOSTING TIP #30: Arm your brain against the effects of long-term stress by eating more seafood, brown rice, almonds, garlic, salmon, flounder, lentils, sunflower seeds, bran, brewer's yeast, and avocados.

BRAIN-BOOSTING TIP #31: Eating the right foods in the right quantities—preferably in the pleasant company of other people—will relieve stress and equip your brain to face distressing challenges.

BRAIN-BOOSTING TIP #32: Snacking on low-carb foods between meals can help to keep blood sugar levels from dipping and affecting your brain-body connection.

BRAIN-BOOSTING TIP #33: Consider juicing certain health-promoting fruits and vegetables to get the nutrients you need to boost your brain as you recover from illness.

BRAIN-BOOSTING TIP #34: Basic good nutrition improves recovery from brain damage that has resulted from the abuse of alcohol or drugs.

BRAIN-BOOSTING TIP #35: If you feel light-headed and dizzy, you might be dehydrated. Boost your brain and get rid of dizziness by drinking more water.

BRAIN-BOOSTING TIP #36: Warm milk induces sleep and helps your brain slow down to be rejuvenated while you rest.

BRAIN-BOOSTING TIP #37: Eat three modest meals and two nutritious snacks every day to start losing weight and boost your brain at the same time.

Brain-Boosting Tip #38: Sprinkle flaxseeds on your oatmeal. They're rich in brain-boosting omega-3 fatty acids.

Brain-Boosting Tip #39: To replenish your brain, increase your serotonin level by eating whole-grain breads or cereals, pasta, potatoes, popcorn, or rice.

Brain-Boosting Tip #40: You can balance your blood sugar and boost your brain's biochemistry by sticking to a low-sugar, high-fiber, and high-protein diet.

Brain-Boosting Tip #41: "Brainy" bedtime snack suggestions include plain yogurt, oatmeal, a small serving of lean turkey, a banana, a small serving of tuna, or a few whole-grain crackers.

Brain-Boosting Tip #42: To keep your brain and body balanced during PMS, eat a high-fiber, high-protein, low-salt, and low-sugar diet.

Brain-Boosting Tip #43: Soybeans, Mexican wild yam, licorice, and black cohosh can help balance a woman's hormones, which leads to better brain health.

Brain-Boosting Tip #44: To balance your brain and your testosterone, increase your intake of zinc-rich foods such as oysters, red meat, and other high-protein foods.

Brain-Boosting Tip #45: Boost your brain with lots of antioxidants found in brightly colored fruits and vegetables.

Brain-Boosting Tip #46: Eat fresh seafood at least twice weekly to help minimize the effects of aging on your brain.

Brain-Boosting Tip #47: Eat a good breakfast every single day for optimum brain function.

Brain-Boosting Tip #48: Dairy products, poultry, fish, lean meats, brown rice, nuts, eggs, legumes, and breads and cereals made with enriched grains supply both niacin and protein, which will give you a better outlook and more energy.

Brain-Boosting Tip #49: Know your own brain and body, and learn how to meet your personal nutritional needs as well as your needs for exercise and rest.

Brain-Boosting Tip #50: Substitute as many brain-boosting foods into your diet as you can for improved brain function and overall health.

NOTES

Chapter 1
How We're Made 101

1. George J. Siegel, ed., *Basic Neurochemistry: Molecular, Cellular and Medical Aspects*, 6th edition (Philadelphia: Lippincott-Raven for the American Society for Neurochemistry, 1999), from chapter 33, "Nutrition and Brain Function," by Gary E. Gibson and John P. Blass, http://www.ncbi.nlm.nih.gov/books/bv.fcgi?rid=bnchm .chapter.2389 (accessed August 20, 2007).

Chapter 2
From the Womb...

1. Womenshealth.gov, "What to Eat When Pregnant," U.S. Department of Health and Human Services, Office on Women's Health, http://womenshealth.gov/pregnancy/pregnancy/eat.cfm (accessed August 20, 2007).

2. Ibid.

3. Ibid.

Chapter 3
Child's Play

1. "Rethinking the Brain—New Insights Into Early Development," Conference Report—Brain Development in Young Children: New Frontiers for Research, Policy and Practice, Organized by the Families and Work Institute, June 1996, National Association of Child Care Resource and Referral Agencies, Washington, DC, http://www1.dshs.wa.gov/pdf/publications/22-300.pdf (accessed January 18, 2008).

2. American Pregnancy Association, "What's in Breast Milk?" http://www.americanpregnancy.org/firstyearoflife/ whatsinbreastmilk.html (accessed August 20, 2007).

3. National Food Service Management Institute fact sheet, "What's Cooking?" Volume 4, Number 4, University of Mississippi, posted by the New York State Department of Health at http://www.health .state.ny.us/prevention/nutrition/resources/baby.htm (accessed August 20, 2007).

4. Summarized on Medline Plus, "Infant and Toddler Nutrition," U.S. National Library of Medicine and National Institutes of Health, http://www.nlm.nih.gov/medlineplus/ infantandtoddlernutrition.html (accessed August 21, 2007).

CHAPTER 5
NOURISH YOUR BRAIN: GABA AND MAGNESIUM

1. "GABA," *Supplement News*, http://www.supplementnews.org/ gaba/index.htm (accessed January 18, 2008).

CHAPTER 6
FISH = BRAIN FOOD

1. Harvard School of Public Health, "What Is Protein?" http:// www.hsph.harvard.edu/nutritionsource/protein.html (accessed August 22, 2007).

2. Ibid.

3. The Nutritive Value of Foods, United States Department of Agriculture (USDA), http://www.nal.usda.gov/fnic/foodcomp/Data/ HG72/hg72_2002.pdf (accessed January 18, 2008).

CHAPTER 7
ANTIOXIDANTS AND YOUR BRAIN

1. For more information, see "Understanding Free Radicals and Antioxidants" at http://www.healthchecksystems.com/antioxid.htm.

2. International Food Information Council Foundation, "Functional Foods Fact Sheet: Antioxidants," March 2006, http:// www.ific.org/publications/factsheets/antioxidantfs.cfm (accessed August 24, 2007).

3. Medline Plus, "Antioxidants," U.S. National Library of Medicine and National Institutes of Health, http://www.nlm.nih.gov/ medlineplus/antioxidants.html (accessed August 24, 2007).

CHAPTER 8
WATER: PURE AND ESSENTIAL

1. Kristen D'Anci, Florence Constant, Irwin Rosenberg, "Hydration and Cognitive Function in Children," *Nutrition Reviews* 64, 2006, http://www.ars.usda.gov/research/publications/ Publications.htm?seq_no_115=201750 (accessed January 16, 2008).

CHAPTER 12
ALL-IMPORTANT NEUROTRANSMITTERS

1. Candace Pert, "Emotional Stress Leads to Immune Suppression," *Prevention Magazine*, April 1994, 73–79.

2. Fran Berkoff, "Can Foods Boost Your Mood?" CanadianLiving .com, http://www.canadianliving.com/CanadianLiving/client/en/ today/DetailNews.asp?idNews=237096&bSearch=True (accessed August 21, 2007).

CHAPTER 13
EMOTIONAL DISORDERS

1. "Common Symptoms of Panic Attacks," The Linden Center, Nampa, Idaho, http://www.panic-anxiety.com/panic_attack_ symptoms/panic-attack-symptoms.htm. Accessed August 24, 2007.

CHAPTER 14
FOR YOUR MOODS: "DO" AND "DON'T" FOODS

1. Anna Delany, "What's Your Food Doing for Your Mood?" Calorie King Library, http://www.calorieking.com/library/articles/ Whats-Your-Food-Doing-for-Your-Mood_YWlkPTg5Ng.htm (accessed August. 21, 2007).

2. Charles Stuart Platkin, "Change in Your Mood? It Just Might Be Your Food," *The Honolulu Advertiser*, July 16, 2003, http://the .honoluluadvertiser.com/article/2003/Jul/16/il/il07a (accessed August 10, 2007).

3. Ibid.

4. Suggestions taken from results of The Food and Mood Project survey, a study undertaken in Great Britain with the support of a Millennium Award from Mind, a mental health charity in the United Kingdom, and the Cyril Cordon Trust. Survey results at www.foodandmood.org/Pages/sh-survey.html. The Food and Mood Project, P. O. Box 2737, Lewes, East Sussex, BN7 2GN, UK.

CHAPTER 17
EATING DISORDERS AND YOUR BRAIN

1. Medline Plus, "Eating Disorders," U.S. National Library of Medicine and National Institutes of Health, http://www.nlm.nih .gov/medlineplus/eatingdisorders.html (accessed August 24, 2007).

2. "Seeking Treatment," National Eating Disorders Association, http://www.nationaleatingdisorders.org/p.asp?WebPage_ID=295 (accessed August 24, 2007).

CHAPTER 18
TOO TIRED TO THINK STRAIGHT?
MAYBE IT'S YOUR DIET.

1. "Special Diets for Food Allergies," Cleveland Clinic Foundation health information resources, http://www.clevelandclinic.org/ health/health-info/docs/2900/2987.asp?index=10014 (accessed August 24, 2007).

CHAPTER 19
WHAT DOES FOOD HAVE TO DO WITH IT?

1. C. B. Gesch et al., "Influence of Supplementary Vitamins, Minerals and Essential Fatty Acids on the Antisocial Behaviour of Young Adult Prisoners: Randomised, Placebo-Controlled Trial," *British Journal of Psychiatry* 181 (2002): 22–28, as cited in Reeta Hakkarainen (Department of Mental Health and Alcohol Research, National Public Health Institute, Helsinki, Finland) et al., "Food and Nutrient Intake in Relation to Mental Wellbeing," *Nutrition Journal* 3 (2004): 14, online at PubMed Central, National Library of Medicine, National Institutes of Health, http://www.pubmedcentral .nih.gov/articlerender.fcgi?artid=519023#B3 (accessed August 24, 2007).

2. A. Neumeister et al., "Effects of Tryptophan Depletion in Fully Remitted Patients With Seasonal Affective Disorder During Summer," *Psychological Medicine* 28 (1998): 257–264, as cited in Hakkarainen et al., "Food and Nutrient Intake in Relation to Mental Wellbeing."

3. Hakkarainen et al., "Food and Nutrient Intake in Relation to Mental Wellbeing."

4. L. M. Bodnar, "Nutrition and Depression," *Biological Psychiatry* 58, no. 9 (November 1, 2005)): 679–685, online at PubMed Central, National Library of Medicine, National Institutes of Health, http://www.ncbi.nlm.nih.gov/sites/entrez?cmd=Retrieve&db=PubMed&list_uids=16040007&dopt=AbstractPlus (accessed August 24, 2007).

Chapter 21
Migraines and Other Headaches Eating You Up?

1. Summarized on Medline Plus, "Migraine," U.S. National Library of Medicine and National Institutes of Health, http://www.nlm.nih.gov/medlineplus/migraine.html (accessed January 21, 2008). Information supplied by The National Institute of Neurological Disorders and Stroke.

2. "Migraine Headaches," University of Maryland Medical Center, Complementary and Alternative Medicine index, http://www.umm.edu/altmed/articles/migraine-headache-000072.htm (accessed January 21, 2008). Information supplied by the American Accreditation HealthCare Commission (A.D.A.M.), copyright 2003.

Chapter 22
Strokes and Transient Ischemic Attacks: The Nutrition Link

1. Information from Medline Plus, U.S. National Library of Medicine and National Institutes of Health, "Transient Ischemic Attack," http://www.nlm.nih.gov/medlineplus/transientischemicattack.html (accessed August 27, 2007), and "Stroke," http://www.nlm.nih.gov/medlineplus/stroke.html (accessed August 27, 2007).

2. Summarized from "Transient Ischemic Attacks," University
of Maryland Medical Center, Complementary and Alternative
Medicine index, http://www.umm.edu/altmed/articles/transient
-ischemic-000160.htm#Treatment%20Options (accessed August 27,
2007), and "Stroke," http://www.umm.edu/altmed/articles/stroke
-000159.htm (accessed August 27, 2007). Information supplied by
the American Accreditation HealthCare Commission (A.D.A.M.),
copyright 2004 and 2006.

3. Jean Carper, "Boost Your Brain," *USA Weekend*, March 5, 2000,
http://www.usaweekend.com/00_issues/000305/000305eatsmart
.html (accessed January 17, 2008).

CHAPTER 23
INFLAMMATION AND NUTRITION

1. Information taken from Michael Downey, "The Battle Within:
Our Anti-Inflammation Diet," *Better Nutrition*, February 2005,
http://betternutrition.richard-group.com/document/633 (accessed
August 27, 2007).

CHAPTER 25
THYROID DYSFUNCTION AND YOUR DIET

1. "Hypothyroidism" and "Hyperthyroidism," University of
Maryland Medical Center, Complementary and Alternative
Medicine index, http://www.umm.edu/altmed/articles/
hypothyroidism-000093.htm (accessed August 27, 2007), and
http://www.umm.edu/altmed/articles/hyperthyroidism-000088.htm
(accessed August 27, 2007). Information supplied by the American
Accreditation HealthCare Commission (A.D.A.M.), copyright 2006.

CHAPTER 26
OVERCOMING CHRONIC FATIGUE SYNDROME

1. "Charles Lapp, MD, on the Effective Treatment of Chronic
Fatigue Syndrome and Fibromyalgia," ProHealth, ImmuneSupport
.com, http://www.immunesupport.com/library/showarticle.cfm/
id/3942 (accessed January 21, 2008).

CHAPTER 27
FIGHTING OFF FIBROMYALGIA

1. Thomas Fisher, "Fibromyalgia," Discovery Health, http://health
.discovery.com/encyclopedias/illnesses.html?article=648 (accessed
January 21, 2008).

2. National Fibromyalgia Association, FibroHOPE, "Seven Lifestyle
Tips," http://www.fibrohope.org/fibromyalgia_lifestyle_tips.asp
(accessed January 21, 2008).

CHAPTER 28
CONQUERING CHRONIC PAIN

1. Orthopod, "Chronic Pain and Nutrition," August 14, 2007,
http://www.eorthopod.com/public/patient_education/7458/
chronic_pain_and_nutrition.html (accessed January 21, 2008).

CHAPTER 29
NOURISHING THE OVERTAXED BRAIN

1. Kari Watson, "The Brain's Balancing Act," *Natural Health*,
September/October 1998.

2. Linda Rector Page, "Personality Perils of Sugar," *Healthy
Healing*, 11th Edition (n.p.: Traditional Wisdom, Inc., 2000), 170.

CHAPTER 30
WHAT HAS STRESS DONE TO YOUR BRAIN?

1. Your Amazing Brain, "Stress: Your Brain and Body," http://www
.youramazingbrain.org/brainchanges/stressbrain.htm (accessed
January 17, 2008).

CHAPTER 32
UNDOING PSYCHOSOMATIC KNOTS

1. "Mind-Body Medicine—an Overview," National Center for
Complementary and Alternative Medicine, National Institutes of
Health, http://nccam.nih.gov/health/backgrounds/mindbody
.htm#ref (accessed September 5, 2007).

CHAPTER 33
THINKING THROUGH TO HEALTH:
RECOVERY FROM A MAJOR ILLNESS

1. American Cancer Society, "Making Treatment Decisions/Diet
and Nutrition," http://www.cancer.org/docroot/eto/eto_5_2_2
.asp?sitearea=eto (accessed September 5, 2007).

CHAPTER 34
REPAIRING DAMAGE FROM DRUGS OR ALCOHOL

1. C. S. Lieber, "The Influence of Alcohol on Nutritional Status,"
Nutrition Reviews 46, no. 7 (1988): 241–254, as quoted in "Alcohol
Alert," National Institute on Alcohol Abuse and Alcoholism No. 22
PH 346, October 1993. All material contained in the Alcohol Alert
is in the public domain and may be used or reproduced without
permission from NIAAA. Complete document is available from
the Scientific Communications Branch, Office of Scientific Affairs,
NIAAA, 5600 Fishers Lane, Room 16C-14, Rockville, MD 20857.

2. M. A. Korsten, "Alcoholism and Pancreatitis: Does Nutrition
Play a Role?" *Alcohol Health & Research World* 13, no. 3 (1989):
232–237, as quoted in "Alcohol Alert."

3. Ibid. Also L. Feinman and C. S. Lieber, "Nutrition: Medical
Problems of Alcoholism," in C. S. Lieber, ed., *Medical and
Nutritional Complications of Alcoholism: Mechanisms in
Management* (New York: Plenum Publishing Corp., 1992) 515–530,
as quoted in "Alcohol Alert."

4. Korsten, "Alcoholism and Pancreatitis: Does Nutrition Play a
Role?" *Alcohol Health & Research World* 13, no. 3 (1989): 232–237,
as quoted in "Alcohol Alert."

5. Lieber, "The Influence of Alcohol on Nutritional Status." Also
C. S. Lieber, "Alcohol and Nutrition: An Overview," *Alcohol Health
& Research World* 13, no. 3 (1989): 197–205, as quoted in "Alcohol
Alert."

6. Ibid. Also M. A. Leo and C. S. Lieber, "Alcohol and Vitamin A,"
Alcohol Health & Research World 13, no. 3 (1989): 250–254, as
quoted in "Alcohol Alert."

7. Ibid.

8. E. B. Flink, "Magnesium Deficiency in Alcoholism," *Alcoholism: Clinical and Experimental Research* 10, no. 6 (1986): 590–594, as quoted in "Alcohol Alert."

9. L. Marsano and C. J. McClain, "Effects of Alcohol on Electrolytes and Minerals," *Alcohol Health & Research World* 13, no. 3 (1989): 255–260, as quoted in "Alcohol Alert."

10. C. J. McClain et al., "Zinc Metabolism in Alcoholic Liver Disease," *Alcoholism: Clinical and Experimental Research* 10, no. 6 (1986): 582–589, as quoted in "Alcohol Alert."

11. "Alcohol and Nutrition—A Commentary by NIAAA Director Enoch Gordis, MD" from "Alcohol Alert."

12. Statement for the Record of Alan I. Leshner, PhD, Director, National Institute on Drug Abuse, before the Senate Governmental Affairs Committee, Monday, July 30, 2001. Department of Health and Human Services, National Institutes of Health, Washington DC.

CHAPTER 38
BRAIN BALANCERS

1. Joseph Hibbeln, MD, lead clinical investigator for the National Institute on Alcohol Abuse and Alcoholism, Bethesda, Maryland. Informational pamphlet.

CHAPTER 39
REPLENISH YOUR BRAIN

1. Fran Berkoff, "Can Foods Boost Your Mood?" CanadianLiving .com, http://www.canadianliving.com/CanadianLiving/client/en/ today/DetailNews.asp?idNews=237096&bSearch=True (accessed August 21, 2007).

CHAPTER 43
HORMONAL HARMONY: MENOPAUSE

1. From the "Healthy Menopause Diet—15 Suggestions," Anne Collins Weight Loss Program, http://www.annecollins.com/best -diet-for-menopause.htm (accessed September 13, 2007).

2. Ibid.

CHAPTER 44
HORMONAL HARMONY: ANDROPAUSE
("MALE MENOPAUSE")

1. K. T. Brill et al., "Single and Combined Effects of Growth Hormone and Testosterone Administration on Measures of Body Composition, Physical Performance, Mood, Sexual Function, Bone Turnover, and Muscle in Healthy Older Men," *The Journal of Clinical Endrocrinology and Metabolism* 87 (December 2002): 5649–5657.

2. Title unknown, *Science* (September 1984): 1032–1034.

CHAPTER 45
B IS FOR BRAIN-BOOSTING

1. Rosalie Marion Bliss, "Nutrition and Brain Function," *Agricultural Research*, August 2007, reprinted on the Agricultural Research Service (United States Department of Agriculture) at http://www.ars.usda.gov/is/AR/archive/aug07/aging0807.htm (accessed September 13, 2007).

2. Ibid.

3. Information taken from The Nutritive Value of Foods, United States Department of Agriculture (USDA).

CHAPTER 47
ENERGY TO SPARE

1. Elizabeth Somer, *Food & Mood*, as quoted by Platkin, "Change in Your Mood? It Just Might Be Your Food."

2. Information taken from The Nutritive Value of Foods, United States Department of Agriculture (USDA).

3. "Protein," Harvard School of Public Health, http://www.hsph .harvard.edu/nutritionsource/protein.html (accessed September 13, 2007).

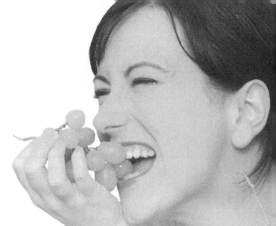

YOUR MOODS & EMOTIONS
CAN ROB YOU OF A
Happy, Healthy Life

We hope you have discovered new ways to sharpen your mind through the foods you eat with *Brain-Boosting Foods*. Here is another book by Dr. Janet that will put you on the road to better health today!

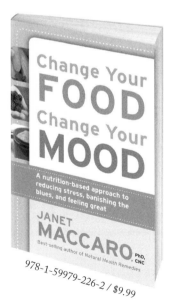

978-1-59979-226-2 / $9.99

Proper nutrition can balance and repair brain chemistry —without drugs—and the results can be felt within minutes. Dr. Janet Maccaro explains the connection, providing a clear list of dos and don'ts that will help you relieve stress, anger, depression, and more.

Experience better health in all areas of your life today!

Visit your local bookstore.

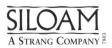

A STRANG COMPANY

7803

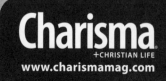